ONE MAN'S JOURNEY THROUGH THE NURSING LIFE,
A PERSONAL ACCOUNT OF THE HIGHS AND LOWS

OH, NURSE!

David Daniels, RN

Publishing Services provided by Paper Raven Books

Printed in the United States of America

First Printing, 2019

Paperback ISBN= 978-0-578-44265-5
Hardback ISBN= 978-0-578-44266-2

Dedicated in loving memory of Colleen Mahoney, RN (RIP),
the finest emergency department nurse I've ever known

"We can do no great things, only small things with great love."

—Mother Teresa

TABLE OF CONTENTS

PREFACE

Nursing has many stories, but this one is mine. I have attempted to provide the reader a glimpse of what my own personal experience has been. The emergency department presents cases spontaneously, often with very little warning. Patients arrive either by the front door or the ambulance entrance. Then the nurse reacts to what is; the who, what, when, where, and why factor very little, if at all. You, the reader, may have a difficult time finding any direction or continuity, because the pace may seem quick and, well, the ER is chaotic. I can only hope I adequately reflected all of that. What you follow is my nursing career from the beginning to nearly the end.

Nursing, I feel, is a most sacred profession. It is the nurse who holds the very fabric of society and patients' medical care together, always keeping an ever-watchful eye, representing true caring. Nursing is both a science and what I've learned is most certainly an art; the nurse will think with the mind and act with the heart.

In my time, I've also come to recognize that almost anyone can get through nursing school and receive their RN, but not everyone will become a nurse.

This book has been inspired by actual events and therefore, by varying degrees, stories have been fictionalized. In order to maintain respect and privacy of individuals both living and dead, all names have been changed with the exception of one.

THE BEGINNING

I remember walking through the halls of the junior college A group of girls in white uniforms were exiting what appeared to be a lab class, but not just any lab class. As the door swung open, I caught a glimpse of dead bodies. The students were noticeably excited. While I remember thinking that they must be pretty strong to be in there, it didn't occur to me again for some time.

Years later, in between construction projects on the street I was living, the aroma of garlic was wafting into my apartment through the window screen. It was my neighbor, a most delightful Englishwoman who seemed to spend most of her time at home. She was always cooking. Bored, hungry, and curious, I knocked on her door hoping for a sample tasting. I had to ask, "How is it you're home so much?"

In her accent she replied, "I'm a nurse." She worked labor and delivery (L&D), which meant she helped deliver babies at the hospital just down the street.

I was thinking, "I could use a change and do something meaningful with my life— something that counts and that I could be really proud of. Yes! Oh, and of course I could be home all the time, too, which would allow me the time to surf more!"

I met my other neighbor who was a nurse also. I spoke with him about my idea. While I was paging through his copies of *Nursing* magazine, probing for more information on what nursing was like, his only response was, "No! Don't do it." Clearly, he was unhappy.

I bounced my new idea off a very close old friend whose response was, "I just don't see you able to handle dealing with doctors very well! We had a good laugh, and I knew I could prove him wrong.

The very next day, I walked into the hospital down the street. I found the volunteer office and asked if I could volunteer there. I told them I wanted to be in their emergency room, because my aspiration was eventually to become an ER nurse. They were happy to have me and told me I would be starting the following Sunday in the ER!

I showed up that Sunday morning ready for my new ER experience, but I was told there was another young man from the local high school assigned to the emergency department. I was told he wanted to be a doctor. Instead of what I expected to do in the ER, I had to hand out newspapers to patients out on the medical surgery floor. Hmm, I guess the aspiration to become a doctor carried a lot more weight.

As luck (or fate) would have it, a nurse approached me and told me if I volunteered at the county hospital for 40 hours, I would receive a phlebotomy certificate. This meant I could draw blood! I found my way into the basement of this old county hospital, walked into this small room where they were drawing blood, and introduced myself. The next morning, I began my 40-hour experience sticking people with needles, drawing their blood, and trying to remember the correct tubes to collect the blood. All the while, I was being taught by Gloria, a wonderful woman who wore too much lipstick. Her hip was shot, so she would hobble down the halls. She could get blood from anyone, and I remember I was always wiping her lipstick off my face. It was a great time, Gloria and me side by side. After the 40 hours, they hired me. I was in, and my journey had now begun!

The days started at 0600. We would grab our trays and go to the postpartum floor to draw blood from the new mothers. From there, we would move to pediatrics. It was certainly a challenge waking the children by sticking them with needles. It was a task to keep them from out-wrestling me. My eardrums were reverberating for hours while they would scream, cry, and throw up all over me. After heading to the psychiatric department, drawing lithium levels, we would then make our trek back to the outpatient lab, where we would continue blood draws until noon.

Somehow, I became trusted enough to draw the newborns. Most of the time, blood was collected with a heel stick, which basically meant stabbing the heel of the baby and then squeezing the foot until the plastic "bullets" were full. Once in a while, the doctor would order "central," which meant I had to use a needle to make the venipuncture. I was sticking needles into the arms of one-day-old babies.

Eventually, I was assigned to the neonatal unit, which was an ICU for premature infants. This was serious. The nurses there were ever-watchful and would not allow just anyone near their babies. I got in and stayed in! Long before modern advances in pulmonology, these little ones were all on ventilators so alarms constantly beeped. I became so attuned to all the noise, I was able to detect a noise that differed from 17 ventilators that were sounding at the same time. I went over to the desk and hung up the phone.

I liked the NICU, the nurses were great, and the doctors were brilliant. The doctors would round on the babies and say things like, "He has a PDA. This one has PFC, with RLF and BPD." I didn't have a clue as to what they were talking about. It was their own special code. I was learning so much about the babies. One of the doctors grabbed me and had me put an IV line through the baby's umbilical cord. They wanted me to stay and work there once I graduated from nursing school. While the thought was nice, I knew I wanted to become an ER nurse.

CHAPTER 1

WALKING THROUGH NEW DOORS

It all started with nursing school. I had completed the prerequisites: anatomy, physiology, chemistry, and microbiology. These were fascinating subjects, and after each course I wanted to change my major. However, every professor said the same thing, "Stay in nursing, we need good nurses." For some reason, I listened and adhered to their advice.

Nursing school was certainly a different experience. For two years, I had recurring feelings rumbling through my gut. The first was a need to survive and get through it. The other was more of a question: "Why am I being punished?" That question has followed me for 30 years! After all, I just wanted to be a nurse. I was always made to feel like I was doing something wrong.

Ms. Tom was my first instructor. She was wonderful and inspired a great degree of excitement. She taught us how to wash our hands and why. We also learned how to take a blood pressure. Ms. Tom had a special stethoscope that would allow her to listen in at the same time. You had to get it right! All of these skills were easy enough, but some of the students with prior hospital experience went on and on about their patients and their experiences with family. A simple lecture would be followed by tangents of hair-washing and curling, and on and on and on. I would be squirming in my seat, asking, "Can we just get on with the lecture?"

Nursing school was tricky. We were always being evaluated, and not necessarily on our exam scores. Everything about us was being scrutinized. We had to be very quick on the uptake. It was the rule.

My next instructor was Ms. Sue. She was an awesome instructor, capable of inspiring fear in most. She always looked us straight in the eye and walked with her heals clicking, a goose step was more like it. We would definitely hear her coming.

Now, Ms. Sue arranged the patient assignments, and I could tell you that for one year I never had a patient who could talk to me. The other students had patients who could ambulate and take their own showers, but mine were always in a coma. Every morning, I would find them full of shit (FOS). Now, I am not a conspiracy theorist, but I am sure those assignments were intentional and as far as the FOS part, I'm guessing they were a gift from the staff nurse to the student nurse.

At this point, I was the only male nurse in the class. A paramedic was also with me, but he washed out in no time. I remember what he first told me, "If the patient is breathing, there's no emergency. If the breathing stopped, the emergency is over." Maybe that's why he did not last.

Ms. Sue was always around me, and when it was time for any procedure she recruited me. As result, I was getting a ton of experience. I knew she was pushing to see if I really wanted to become a nurse. I never blinked.

One day, I was assigned a nice little old lady. I walked in the room to introduce myself and she did not respond. I stepped closer to find her eyes closed and a blueish-purple color around her neck. She was cool, and her breathing was wrong. I stepped out of the room, and immediately Ms. Sue asked me how I felt about being there. I told her I was fine but asked what exactly she expected me to do. After all, I was just a student. She told me to clean up the woman before her family arrived. As I began to bathe her, two nurses came in and took a box with wires off the lady's chest and then they excused me. That was the first time a patient died in front of me, and I really didn't even know it.

Ms. Sue was right there and asked me how I felt about death. I told her I thought death sucked but that I was familiar with it. I shared with her that some time ago, I'd woken on a particular Monday morning to watch the undertaker take my father away. Again, I didn't blink.

Looking back, Ms. Sue really did right by me. She prepared me, pushed me, and to this day she's still on my shoulder as a voice of conscience! I always use alcohol on the IV hubs because of what she taught me, and as a rule once something hit the floor it stayed there.

School was busy, volumes to read, clinical to prepare for. I had the weekends to decompress, so I would go to my hospital to draw blood and study. There were three other students working the weekends with me. We would share our stories. Karen's were the best! She was a fiery redheaded Irish girl, and I remember a story she told that I'll never forget. One morning, she was feeding a patient who had suffered a stroke and was blind. She was very close to the patient who, unfortunately, had very bad breath. He kept choking on the food, which would roll around between his teeth and gums while he would gag. In no time, she threw up on the patient! I was dying, laughing in tears! She threw up on her patient! Poor man.

I told them about a time I went to draw blood from a patient. He was in traction with two broken legs and needed to pee, but both of his urinals were full to the top. I knew I had to get the nurse, because they might be measuring his urine output. In response, he told me he'd been calling them, but they didn't answer his bell. I found the nurse and told her the patient needed her. She got mad at me, saying "Well your just bound to make me get up!"

I was like, "He's got two broken legs!"

I told them about a different kind of room I visited. The sign said, "reverse isolation," which meant I had to wear a gown, gloves, and mask, because the man's immune system could not fight infection. I went into the room to draw his blood and noticed that he looked especially sick and was very, very thin. He was alone and scared. At that time, no one knew what he had. I told them I thought he was dying. As time went on, there were more men like him on the floor.

Karen then told us she'd walked into a room where the patient's trachea was being suctioned. She was standing at the foot of the bed when the guy coughed a thick wad of sputum that landed on her face! As she tried to remove the sputum, it stuck to her cheek. She threw up on that guy, too!

I was laughing so hard. So as not to one up her, I recited how I was helping clean up a patient who was full of shit. The student was spraying Peri-Wash that bounced off the patient's bottom and all over my face. That was a big thank you!

Soon, I was heading into my last semester. I felt it was time to make some changes if I wanted to become an ER nurse. I was lucky that the ER in the hospital where I worked did hire student nurses! I was able to transfer and work weekends through the rest of the school year and summer. It was then that everything changed! The place was busy, the lights were bright, all kinds of people running everywhere. It appeared in my eyes to be total chaos, but there were some people who looked totally in control and as calm as could be. I was completely out of my element and had no business being in there. It was, well, kind of scary. I found myself standing next to a supply cart and quickly walked away from it for fear someone would ask me to grab something. I was directed to a desk where I would be sitting in between two others. I was safe, or so I thought. The one clerk sat me in the corner, where a tube ran from the desk and up into the ceiling. She showed me how to wrap blood tubes into a canister and send the blood to the lab by way of that tube. I thought it was crazy. I just pushed a button and away the blood went.

Sitting in my safe little corner, I heard a radio alarm go off. It was a paramedic radio. As the nurse answered it, she announced a full arrest was coming. I didn't really know what a full arrest was. It sounded serious and soon I would find out. Immediately, a team assembled in the resuscitation room. The medics arrived. I could see though the door that this was serious business. The patient's heart had stopped beating; he was no longer breathing, so the team went to work! Instantly someone screamed, "We need someone to do CPR!"

The two clerks looked at me, and I at them. They both said, "You're the nursing student." Reluctantly, I walked into the room, stepped up onto this stool, and began chest compressions on this man. Someone was squeezing a bag to breathe for him, drugs were called out, and every once in a while, I would notice a tap on my shoulder. The doctor would tell me to hold CPR, then he would tap me again and say resume CPR. I trusted that voice and only did what he told me. The man died. I helped put a tag on his toe. We zipped him in a plastic bag, rolled him upstairs, logged him in, and slid his body into a big refrigerator. I can still see that man's face today.

Ms. Boyle was my instructor for the psychiatric nursing module. I didn't care too much for it. I liked the energy in the ER and wanted to get back there. One day, I spent the entire shift with a patient who did nothing but mumble and pick his nose. He had a deck of cards, but there was no way I was about to shuffle that deck and start dealing! I finished the rotation easily enough. As it concluded, Ms. Boyd gave us an exit interview. I went in to get my evaluation, which was fine, but Ms. Boyd expressed her concern for me, cautioning that I was headed for an extreme depressive disorder. I responded, "Can I just have my grade, please?" What did she know? She was just a nursing instructor. I never felt she was qualified to predict my future. I got my grade, drove to the beach, and rode some waves!

Ms. Rae, my next instructor, was a lovely woman. I found her professional and approachable, not as strict as the other instructors. I was also growing into my own and felt more comfortable as a nursing student. I was certainly enjoying my clinicals much more.

Near the end of the module, I found Ms. Rae in the nursing lounge. She was alone, and I noticed some tears running down her face. I walked in to be beside her and came to learn it was on this floor where her husband had passed away from colon cancer not too long ago. We sat together. She gathered herself as we spoke. As I got up to leave, she stopped me and offered some advice. She said it was essential to take the time to care and refresh myself because nursing would chew me up and spit me out once there was nothing left of me. I was taken aback, wondering how she could say this to me. I wasn't even out of school and was dedicated to preparing for a new wonderful adventure, of caring for my fellow man. I didn't blink!

It was a busy Saturday in the ER. The beds were full, bells were ringing. The charge nurse was a cute little blonde from over the hill, the rich part of town. I was working with two other clerks from the hood! We had a ball working together. I somehow always had them laughing. While everyone else was stressing, we were at the desk cracking up. These women were tough. It was better to be on their good side, and I most certainly was.

The charge nurse asked the one clerk to break down a chart since the patient was to be admitted. The breakdown required a huge amount of paperwork to be gone through. As the cute little blonde handed over the chart, the clerk threw the entire packet up to the ceiling, saying "You can break that motherfucker down yourself." The floor was covered with hundreds of pieces of paper. I couldn't breathe, I was laughing so hard. I never ever saw anything like it in the workplace, and this was a hospital! The charge nurse just ran off. I'm not sure who picked up the papers. I don't think the charge nurse ever asked the clerk for anything ever again. This place, I came to realize, was crazy, but I loved it and somehow felt I'd found my home. I soon discovered that in school they teach you how it's supposed to be, but at work it is how it is. Rarely do the twain ever meet!

A nurse came and asked me to help her. She had a patient on a gurney covered with dried blood. He had one stab wound into his heart and he was dead. He was 21 years old, and his life was over. I helped put a tag on his toe and zipped him into a big plastic bag.

Wrapping up my last rotation, I was getting pretty excited. My wife and I became parents to a beautiful girl. My mom called one day after I got home from clinical asking how things were going. It was at a weak moment. I told her my life was shit. I was cleaning patients who stooled themselves, I was changing the baby's diaper, and now it was my turn to take a dump. Yes, my whole life was shit!

My last instructor was Ms. Zale. She was crazy. She spent much of our clinical time in a hallway bathroom that she would fill with her cigarette smoke, and she smelled like a bottle of Jack! I found her to be out of her mind, not only that, she had it out for me. She was on my back constantly. She was my last obstacle. I was planning my argument, as I was sure she wanted me out of the program. My grades were good, I was as competent as a student nurse could be. For sure I thought I was headed to the dean's office to begin the defensive argument against her accusations, but somehow, I did my time and survived her. I was done with her. I graduated!

On my last day, walking through the hospital parking lot, another student saw me. She said, "Hey, you look like you're glowing!" I guess I was, my dream was coming true. I was going to become a nurse! I was going to become an ER nurse!

Oddly enough, later that summer Ms. Zale came into the ER to see a family member whom I was assured she drove crazy enough to end up in our psych room. As she saw me, she began to make some negative comments towards me when another nurse informed her I was one of the best students they'd had, and that I'd be hired once I pass boards! That was sweet!

I spent my time working in that ER as a student. All the while, I was studying and becoming well prepared for my board exams. I took the test, passed, and awaited my license! When it came in the mail, I was immediately hired and began my training as an ER nurse.

There was a group of other students who were hired at the same time. We all quickly became friends and began our training together. These were exciting times. We attended lectures from a variety of physicians, surgeons, and nurses. We learned about different types of emergencies and trauma. It was great! We were also paired up with experienced ER nurses throughout our learning process.

It was a quiet Saturday morning. Nothing was happening, then the paramedic radio went off. All of a sudden, teams formed in the resuscitation room and all three beds were readied. I saw a man enter, CPR in progress. They said he was T-boned coming out of a driveway. They cracked his chest, cut it open, and began squeezing his heart. Blood was everywhere! Bed number two was the lady who hit the guy in bed one. She arrived, CPR in progress, they cracked her chest open, too. There was blood everywhere. The woman was nine months pregnant. The doctors performed a crash C-section and did CPR on the baby. Now bed three came in; it was an older man, full arrest, CPR in progress. Everyone died.

I put all the bodies in body bags after tying tags on their toes. I wheeled the bodies to the morgue and slid them into refrigerated bins. As I walked back to the ER, I doubted my decision to do this job. What was I going to tell my wife now? I just couldn't do it. And yet, a voice inside my head said, "You're going to do this, this is what you wanted."

The lectures wrapped up, the time beside my assigned nurse came to an end, and it was my time to be on my own, ready or not! I was an ER nurse with no experience. It was sink or swim, and quite honestly, I was the most dangerous person in that ER! I didn't even know what I didn't know. I had no skill except for drawing blood! It did come in handy, however, and made starting

IVs a lot easier. At least I had that going for me. Still, it was time to learn ACLS—Advanced Cardiac Life Support! I got the unmistakable impression that there was an expectation that the ER nurse would come into the department prepared to work beside the physicians to save lives. I realized that we were a team of experts of whom excellent performance was demanded and nothing less.

CHAPTER 2

SOME THINGS I'VE NEVER SEEN OR HEARD BEFORE

When things are new, it can sometimes take a while to figure out what's normal and what isn't. Still, if you've been alive long enough, you can generally figure out what's right and what's wrong.

I was just coming out of the resuscitation room when a nurse named Dale asked me if I could help her. I was happy to. Dale had been working the ER for a long time, always appeared angry and ready for a fight. It was rumored she had a cocaine problem.

I asked what she needed, and she replied, "Help putting a Foley in a dirtbag." Now, I knew a Foley was a urinary catheter, but I'd never heard the term dirtbag. It turned out the dirtbag was a patient. I saw the man and he seemed nice enough to me; he looked like he could've been my grandfather. As Dale pulled back the sheet, it was revealed that the patient had shit the bed. In response, Dale became irate and started yelling at the poor old man. Nursing in this particular ER was very different from school. After the incident, I wondered how Dale became a nurse.

Dale had a friend Rena, another nurse in the ER. She struck me as an equally angry person. I walked by as she was training a paramedic student. They were receiving a patient from the field who had an IV placed in the middle fold of his arm. Rena told the student that if she ever received a patient with an IV in his arm like that from him, she would rip his balls off and shove them down his throat! You should have seen the look on that young man's face. Some of these nurses were pretty salty.

Later, I saw Dale in the doctor's office screaming at a surgeon. I was so blown away by how cool he remained as she exploded. She was out of control.

Back at the clerk's desk, we always had a good time. There was one clerk, John, who was a flamboyant homosexual with a great sense of humor. He reminded me of the fashion designer in the movie, *Mannequin*. The only thing that bothered me about him was that he would wear the same perfume I bought for my wife. I would beg him to stop using it for fear he would enter my mind during intimate moments with my spouse. He never quit wearing that perfume, dammit!

One time, he was staring this ER resident up and down, flirtatiously licking his lips. The doctor wasn't amused, and he was a big boy from Hawaii. The more pissed he got, the more flirtatious John became. I was dying, begging him to stop before he got killed. Bear in mind, all this is going on in a very busy emergency room!

There was a patient in the back of the ER secured in leather restraints, delusional and hallucinating. John got on the intercom and began speaking to the patient. He was saying he was the devil, telling the patient to kill himself. I could not believe this was going on. As John laughed, I was thinking, "this is so bad!" In no time, the senior resident approached frantically, telling

John that the family was in the room and heard every word. I ran away from that desk, not wanting any part of it. Later, John developed a bad cough and began to lose a lot of weight. I had come to learn he passed away. I was very sad to hear that news, as his smile and laughter always made the day.

Now the main clerk, Blue, was a lady with all kinds of attitude. She literally was straight out of Compton. She was the one who threw the chart up to the ceiling. I could see her answer the phone and repeatedly hang it up. Later, I found out in the daily newspaper that a family was calling around local hospitals trying to locate their loved one. It took three days before they finally discovered we had admitted the patient into our ICU. I remember thinking, you just can't write this stuff. There're the way things are supposed to be and then there's the way things are.

One day, the chairman of the ER was talking with me. To say the least, he was a brilliant man and a man of many hats. He had a very solemn look on his face. He declared, "The problem is that people don't care about themselves. The hospital administration doesn't care, and the county board of supervisors doesn't care. Nobody cares." I was left wondering why he would tell me that, and in fact how could that really be true.

The back of the ER was more or less a holding unit. Back there, intoxicated, combative psych patients would be watched and evaluated. One of the regular nurses was a wonderful black woman about five feet tall. She would come in every morning and scribe Bible verses on the main white board. She was truly a character. I liked her quite a bit. Whenever we would go out to breakfast and she saw my daughter, she would love her up. It was really sweet. I called her the queen. She'd worked in the back of the ER for a lifetime.

One day, she decided to clean out a rickety old wooden desk. She found a buck knife and gave it to me. I was tickled. As she cleaned further, however, she found a paper bag with 10 thousand dollars! It was unclaimed, and after 30 days the money was hers. Somehow, I think those Bible verses paid off.

Now there was Anna, a most wonderful and caring nurse who seemed to be untouched by the chaos in the ER. I was wondering how that could be. She seemed set apart, if you will. If there was any nurse I admired and wanted to emulate, it was Anna. I knew her from a few years back when I was drawing blood in the neonatal unit. We were always friends. One day, she introduced me to her husband. He was a pretty big guy. When we shook hands, he crushed my hand. It hurt badly. I guess he wanted to make some kind of statement.

CHAPTER 3

MAGGOTS AND NEVER TAKE OFF THE SOCKS

A van pulled up in the ambulance entrance and opened the door to let a man out. He appeared to be homeless. He was dirty, and his pants were held up by rope. He had long, gray hair and was unshaven, and he wore a red baseball cap.

At this point, I was the charge nurse in the ER, so I would make bed assignments and help the overall department flow. I directed the man to a room across from the ER and told the nurse working there about the patient. The patient told me he came in because of his head. He lifted his cap and revealed skin cancer infested with hundreds of crawling maggots!

The nurse was new to the ER, though she did have a lot of previous experience. She wore a white dress and looked like an angel. I neglected to inform her of the maggots but did ask her to have the patient remove his cap. I stood by watching as she jumped about 10 feet back. I had a great laugh!

What I learned about maggots is that you never know when they are going to show up! I remember being at the beach with my cousin. I was hungry and bought a big box of raisins. We started clawing into the box only to look at our hands covered in maggots. Dammit! I couldn't help but think of a music album titled *Maggot Brain*.

Anyway, back in the ER I was working with a nurse who has since become a great friend of mine. Jerry was truly born for ER nursing. He lived it, loved it, and proved to be a great inspiration to me. A trauma patient arrived. He was a frequent visitor to our ER and a homeless young man. This time, he presented with severe burns. Apparently, he was keeping warm by standing around a flaming garbage can. Turns out his buddies decided to burn his legs with red hot shovels. So, the trauma team assembled. Jerry, Cory, and I were the assigned nurses. Cory was the recorder nurse, who charted everything at the foot of the bed. Jerry and I proceeded to remove the patient's clothes, and as Jerry ripped off the patient's socks maggots flew all over Cory's nursing notes! She ran out of the room puking! I had a good chuckle and learned never to take off socks! I never blinked.

CHAPTER 4

REGISTRY NURSING IN THE PRIVATE SECTOR

Ever since I began working in health care, my only experience was the inner-city, county-funded hospital. As I gained some experience and confidence, I picked up extra shifts working through a registry. The company would call and ask if I could work when other hospitals had urgent needs for a nurse.

All I knew is what I learned at my hospital. When a trauma patient arrived, a system of care was designed with specific functions for each of the team members to perform. Different nurses would care for the patient. Some would set up equipment and special procedure trays, while another was responsible for documentation. The nurse charged with recording would scribe the trauma assessment and interventions, record the doctor's head-to-toe assessments, keep times, and record lab values.

One of our responsibilities as trauma nurses was to routinely make sure the proper equipment was available and in working order. As I was going through the shelves inspecting the inventory, I began counting the chest tubes (these were tubes the doctor would insert into a patient's chest, most often in the case of a collapsed lung). While doing so, I noticed other chest tubes called trocars. Now, a trocar chest tube had a kind of large spike inside them. I learned that in certain emergencies, a trocar could be used to punch a hole in between the patient's ribs in order to make the tube insertion.

The technique for chest tube insertion often requires the use of a numbing agent. A small incision in the chest wall is made with a scalpel, then the doctor perforates the muscle between the ribs. After inserting a finger in the cavity to inspect the opening, the tube is inserted, secured, and hooked up to suction, helping the collapsed lung to expand. Now, a collapsed lung can cause problems, but a collapsed lung under pressure (air in the chest pushes the lung over) is a real emergency. In those cases, the doctor must act quickly, usually by inserting a large bore needle in the chest to rapidly release the built-up pressure.

One day, I was working out of the registry in a small private hospital with just one doctor. There were no teams of residents, no interns, and no attending physicians watching over the department. It was the single ER doctor's show. The paramedic radio notified us that we were receiving a victim of a motor vehicle collision. Turned out this guy had stolen a car and wrapped it around a telephone pole. He came in on a backboard with a broken left wrist and a broken nose that was bent to the right. The doctor looked over at him and walked away. He didn't say a word to me, so I was left to my own trauma assessment. I proceeded just like I had been used to at the trauma center. Starting at the head, I moved to his neck. The jugular veins were up, his heart rate was elevated, and he was having trouble breathing. Listening to the sound of his breath, I found it was absent on his left side. Looking at his trachea, I saw it was a bit off-center. I knew immediately that he was developing tension pneumothorax. With his lung collapsed and his heart shifting over to the right side kicking major blood vessels, oxygen delivery, gas exchange, and blood return to the heart were all impeded.

I needed to alert the physician, but how? It was clear he didn't want to be bothered. After all, he was the doctor, I'm just a registry nurse. So, I cautiously approached him and asked if he had listened to the patient's lung sounds (knowing he had not). He replied, "They were a little diminished on the right!"

I responded by noting, "Really, I thought they were a little diminished on the left." I knew the patient didn't have much time and would die if we didn't act. Thankfully, the doctor did get up and walked over to the patient.

He quickly recognized the emergency. To my surprise, rather than sticking the patient with a 16-gauge needle over the top of the third rib in the midclavicular line, he called an in-house surgeon. I watched the older surgeon grab a trocar and slam the chest tube into the patient without anesthesia, much like he was driving home a railroad spike. That kid let out a blood-curdling scream! The pressure was released, and he was able to breathe again! His life was saved!

Now, I was grateful I had learned an adequate trauma assessment and was instrumental in saving this young man's life. At the same time, I could not help but get the feeling that there wasn't much love for African American kids who steal cars in this place. I never experienced that kind of indifference where I worked. I was proud of that fact. I thought that maybe registry stuff is just not for me. I had a co-worker always tell me he would never work in the private sector. I couldn't understand what he meant until now.

CHAPTER 5

ASSIGNED TO TRIAGE AND YOU DON'T WANT TO BE FIRST

The hospital was busy and being placed in the triage booth came with a lot of responsibility. It was certainly not without its challenges, but they were challenges of a different sort.

Triage, I learned, was French meaning "to sort." So being in triage meant sorting out patients by their severity. I listened to the chief complaint of the patient, learned their medical and surgical histories, determined the medication regimen, and took their vital signs. The patient was then prioritized by number. Number one meant critical, two meant emergent, three meant urgent, all the way down to five.

When I said busy, I meant busy. The waiting room was the size of a large movie theatre. A patient was triaged every three to five minutes, constantly, for an entire eight-hour shift! The average wait time was almost twelve hours. Ironically, the patients with a one or two score could not wait and often left without being seen, but the fives could stay and camp out forever! So, the sickest people often never got treated. Eventually, a few doctors gathered data, recognized what was happening, and restructured the system. We became much more effective in seeing the sicker patients as a result.

I always tried to be very sensitive and considerate with the people I triaged, informing them about the time frames, how long they could expect to be waiting. As a result, I didn't have many confrontations. Patients were always invited to come back up to me if anything changed. My co-worker in the next booth, on the other hand, was always getting into shouting matches. The interactions spun out of control, resulting in an eventual call to security. They would proceed to do their thing, often beating the patient into some degree of compliance. I could never understand why she escalated those situations. Apparently, she wanted to establish some sort of dominating control, as if there ever was any.

One time, a sweet little old lady came back up to me. I re-evaluated her and told her that there were still no beds. A while later, she returned, and she was not urgent. I again apologized for the wait and explained there was no place for her at this time. I told her that patients were constantly coming in through our ambulance entrance on the other side of the wall. She was nice enough but looked at me as if she didn't believe me. In fact, she said, "I don't believe you."

I offered to bring her back there, and if she found a spot, it was hers. We walked through the doors and I directed her to the trauma bay. All three beds were full. In bed one, a patient was naked, unresponsive, and on a ventilator. The lady took one look and said, "I'm not that sick."

She instantly wanted to go back out to the waiting room. I held her hand and said, "No, let's keep going, maybe there's a bed for you down the hall." She jerked her hand free, ran to the waiting room, and I didn't see her again for the rest of the shift. Trust me when I say that you don't want to be first in the ER!

As a triage nurse, I gained a variety of skills. One was managing the waiting room and the other was discerning who needed to get back in the ER for immediate medical care. There was no room for mistakes. I also learned that if you made an enemy out of your triage nurse, it would not end up in your favor.

CHAPTER 6

IT'S NOT SUPPOSED TO BE LIKE THIS

Linda was a new nurse in the ER who had an esteemed reputation. Not only was she at the top of her class, but she was also the acting president of the student body, whatever that meant. I clearly received the impression she was "it" as far as ER nursing went.

Our relationship was strained almost instantly. I think it is fair to say she didn't care for me too much. Why? One day, a man came in the ER in a full arrest. We were doing our usual chest compressions, IV, epinephrine, and preparation to defibrillate when Linda said, "Wait, I'm getting a blood pressure."

My tone probably wasn't appreciated when I responded, "Don't worry about his blood pressure right now since he doesn't have a pulse!" So much for being "it."

Later, I had a patient receiving IV fluids and antibiotics, once completed he was to be discharged home. Before completion of the infusions the charge nurse came over to the patient and took out his IV because next to his name on the board it said "home."

When I saw this, I told her to look up! The fluids and antibiotics weren't finished! They were hanging from the pole that was suspended from the ceiling. She laughed at me, as always, and told me to give the patient and the report to Linda. I told Linda that the patient needed the fluids and medicine and explained what the charge nurse had done. Moments later, I saw that Linda sent the man home, no medication, no fluid. I never cared for her much after that.

I had an empty bed and was preparing to receive a patient from down the hall. The nurse who was caring for him had him in a bed in her section for two hours. I could see from the order sheet that nothing was done. The patient had what we call a polydrug overdose. I couldn't believe my eyes. But then it all made sense. The nurse in question was known for refusing to work on patients with AIDS. Accordingly, she'd refused to touch this guy.

Now the irony of her behavior was that she was screwing almost every doctor in the place. She had a particular affinity for trauma surgeons and made sure everyone knew that particular detail. There were times I would walk by a room off to the side of the main ER and find her spraying perfume up her dress, between her legs. I guess she was preparing for her lunch break!

I also noticed that she always wore gloves and never took them off the whole shift. I wondered if she wore gloves when she went home to shower.

Anyway, I looked at the order sheet and told her that what she'd done, or not done, was pure negligence. She began to shout, "Fuck you" and put her middle finger in my face. I asked her three times to move her finger out of my eye, to which she kept screaming "Fuck you." I finally told her I would move her hand myself. She didn't, I did.

Moments later, I found myself in the department manager's office. At times, I've seen people being put on the defensive in these situations, but my manager wasn't that way. Tira was great. We spoke, and all the while she gathered information. She asked me what had occurred. I detailed the time frames, the orders, and what I felt was negligent. Then I described the profanity with the finger thrusted in my eye, followed by my request that it be removed three times, resulting in my eventual decision to move it myself. Tira responded, "I asked the nurse what was wrong with her, invading a man's personal space like that." I thanked Tira and went back to work. She was the best manager I ever had. A few years later, I came to learn Tira was murdered. Such a sad, sad thing.

Chrissy was another nurse, or I guess that's what you'd call her. She wasn't really there to work. The job was more of a social time than anything else for her. She flirted with anyone and everyone. It was well known which doctor she was doing. At times, she'd even take patients home for…. Often, she squeezed herself into tight white jeans with no underwear. Believe me, it was obvious. She hung out at the main desk, posed with her butt out, and did a fine job of arousing the guys in the department. One might say it pays to advertise.

One day, she was looking after an older man who was severely anemic and needed a blood transfusion. I guess he wasn't getting along very well with Chrissy and was refusing her care (not that she cared). He was moved over to my bed, I introduced myself, he seemed nice enough, like someone's grandpa. I explained what we needed to do, and he agreed. I gathered all the supplies and was about to start the IV when he decided he didn't want it. I informed the doctor the patient was now refusing care, he then consulted with the psychiatric department. It was decided the patient was not making a sound decision and was a danger to himself, so I was ordered to put the man in leather restraints and begin the transfusion. I brought over the big hospital bed and asked him to slide off the gurney and onto the bed. The man refused to move, so I told him I would have to move him. I gathered the man in my arms and placed him in the hospital bed. When I let him out of my arms, he was dead. I began CPR but was ordered to stop, so I tagged his toe, zipped him up in a body bag, and wheeled him to the morgue.

On the other side of the main ER was a sort of clinic. Doctors were assigned to see patients who were more or less nonurgent. The wait was longer for obvious reasons. Evidently, a doctor saw a patient who complained about not having seen anyone for hours. The doctor noticed that the patient had his vital signs recorded just a few minutes ago, but the patient said it never happened. Well, as it turned out, the nurse charted vital signs on all the patients who were waiting without ever seeing them! Action was taken, and the nurse was relieved of duty. It's just not supposed to be like this!

The paramedic radio alarmed, we were getting a trauma patient. The ambulance was at the back door in no time at all and chaos broke out. A young man in his late 20s was unresponsive from obvious head trauma. What I could see were clearly defined boot prints all over his head from what looked like hiking boots. He was intubated immediately, but now needed CPR. We worked frantically on him. The story was that his wife was in labor upstairs, and he had just stepped outside to get a newspaper to commemorate the birthday of his child. An argument broke out, resulting in a physical altercation. He died. His wife was a widow and his child was now born without a father. I tagged and bagged the young man and up to the morgue he went.

Another trauma arrived, a young man on a backboard and in a neck collar. He was drunk and had crashed his car. I went over to place him on a heart monitor and got his blood pressure. He spat right in my face. I wiped the spit off and he spat on me again. I remembered Anna, the nurse who always seemed like an angel, and my desire to be like her. Needless to say, it was proving more difficult than I had anticipated. By this point, it had been about five years since I first started nursing. Now I began to wonder how much longer I could last.

CHAPTER 7

A TRIP TO PEDIATRICS

I was getting the run of the ER, I was now seasoned. In reality, just about everyone is seasoned after six months' time in that place. I clocked in and checked my assignment on the board by the nurse manager's office. There was something going on. One of the nurses was in tears. What could have happened? We'd not even started our shift yet!

Suddenly, it was obvious. The nurse had been assigned to the pediatric emergency room. She was crying because she didn't want to go over there. You see, on the adult side, she was often in charge, which meant she could be in front of the resident physicians flirting all day. She was another young lady who spent her time washing her hair with fragrant shampoos, doing her makeup, and wearing the tight white jeans—standard dress code for the female ER nurses who were looking to arouse and perhaps snag the vulnerable young doctors. It was the PM shift, and it was show time! She had to be front stage center! I would often wonder if some of these women went into nursing because of a "calling" or to increase their probability of marrying a doctor? Hmmm.

Now, I didn't work in pediatrics nor did I have any desire to. With young children at home, I thought it would be too difficult for me emotionally. However, there was a need, so I sucked it up and went over there. Not knowing what to expect, I dove right in.

After some time in there, the pediatric ER was the only place I wanted to be. I met one nurse who was awesome. We clicked immediately. There were also a clerk and a technician. We became great friends. The place was busy, and I was learning a lot. Those early years of phlebotomy really paid off. I could get blood and start IVs without a problem. If I couldn't get an IV, my colleague Kate could. If Kate couldn't, I could. We were a formidable team. I learned a lot from the doctors in pediatrics. It was great. I was never prouder of what I did for work! I was becoming a pediatric ER nurse.

I believe in angels, and I met another one. She had blond hair and was pure as newly fallen snow. Mary completed her residency in emergency medicine and stayed on staff as faculty. She was an attending physician and focused on pediatric emergency medicine. She was brilliant, focused, driven, and had a way of communicating that was awe-inspiring. She was always educating, and I would hang on every word. Without exaggeration, I can say that being in her presence made me want to become a better nurse. I could think of no one else I desired to get an affirmative nod from more. Her work transformed pediatric emergency medicine throughout the state and she shaped prehospital care for children as well.

As time went on, she pushed me to become a PALS instructor, which stands for Pediatric Advanced Life Support. I don't know what she saw in me, but I always followed her lead. I was beginning to teach the new interns airway management and resuscitation. The more I got to teach, the more I got to learn as well. It was awesome. Truly, I believe that if I've done any good in my nursing career, it was a result of being in Mary's presence. I'm eternally grateful to her. We had a ball in pediatrics. There was a lot of positive energy. It was very different than all the violent trauma, drug overdoses, and the like on the adult side. We were helping children, we were often saving their lives.

An intercom in the nurse's station reached both the adult and pediatric waiting rooms, even out to the parking lot. During the holidays, I sang "I'll Be Home for Christmas" in my best Elvis voice. Everyone was in tears, laughing. I never got in trouble, and I never stopped my singing. I loved that place. I was on stage, kinda!

Headed out the door one Christmas Eve after finishing my PM shift, the shift supervisor caught me and asked me to work a double. Apparently, they were short on nights. I thought, "Come on, it's Christmas Eve. A double?!" I wanted to get back to my kids, my family. I had bikes to assemble and gifts to wrap and get under the tree!

But I'm soft and have a hard time saying no, so I agreed to do only half the shift. As I returned to the pediatrics ER, the paramedic radio alarmed. We were getting a full cardiac arrest. The patient was an eight-year-old girl. The story was she was vomiting and had diarrhea for quite some time. She couldn't replace her fluid loss, which resulted in hypovolemic shock. She succumbed to decompensated shock, leading to cardiovascular collapse and now arrested. We learned that earlier, the parents took her to their doctor, who prescribed some kind of suppository. With no improvement, the father called the doctor back and who directed them to bring the child back in for a second visit. She arrested in her father's arms on the way to the car. They called 911, and the girl was transported to my ER. We worked on her feverishly, we were not successful. We could not resuscitate her she did not survive. I was thinking if only she came here to this ER first, she might be alive, in fact I would have bet on it.

I spent the remainder of that shift, and what was left of the eight-hour night, with that mother and father. By morning, I escorted them to their car, with only each other—that's all they had. Somehow, I helped them get to the point where they could leave the hospital without their little girl. That was my strongest nursing moment up to that point. I was ready to get back home to my family and celebrate Christmas. Christmas morning was going to be just a little sweeter for me. I hugged my babies just a little longer, just a little tighter.

Back to work, it was business as usual. We saw a lot of pediatric fevers. Since most of the population was at the bottom rung of the socioeconomic ladder, the kids got a full workup. Included in the workup were blood draws, a catheter urine specimen, a chest x-ray, and a lumbar puncture. The doctors looked anywhere and everywhere for infection. These kids got good care. At times, the indications may have been questionable, but after all it was a training ground for the new and soon-to-be doctors. We always sent the family's home with antibiotics, antipyretics, formula, and diapers. They were truly cared for.

In the midst of our workload, the shift supervisor asked me to clean out some storage shelves in the crash room. They were planning some remodeling there, so I told her I would get after it. During the shift, we had two cardiac arrests. Two kids came in separately. We worked furiously but had no success. They both died. I tagged them and bagged them and up to the morgue they went. The shift was over, the staff was spent, and we went home.

I returned the next day and the same shift supervisor approached me, she was licking her chops. She couldn't wait to tear into me for refusing to follow her instructions given the previous day. I asked her, "Do you even know what happened last night?" Now, this was the same lady who begged me to work overtime Christmas Eve!

I remembered my old nursing instructor: "Nursing will chew you up and spit you out when there's nothing left of you!" I just looked at her. I never blinked. I began to realize that while nurses care for everyone no one cares about nurses. I had dealt with two dead children and was present for their grieving families, instead of being acknowledged for my nursing role or even asked if I was okay, I was reprimanded, I was being punished!

Walking back into the department, I was now informed we were getting two kids injured in a house fire. Upon arrival it was clear they were about two and three years old, respectively. The ER resident was new, it was her first day running the department. I looked at the kids, saw their faces which were red and blistered, and began to gather supplies. It was obvious they were going to need immediate attention. I saw the resident leave the room, so I chased her down and asked, "Aren't you going to intubate these kids?" She asked me why she should, immediately I responded, "If I were you, I would tube them while you still have the chance!" Once in a while, a doctor will listen to a nurse, and it's usually a very good thing. Sometimes those little minute things, those slight nudges, make a good doctor a great one.

Without delay, we opened the intubation tray. She viewed the airway with a laryngoscope and placed the tube in the trachea of one of the children. Once it was secured, we moved onto the other child. Afterwards, the doctor approached me and said, "Thank you so much for pushing me. How did you know?" All I said was I read a book from a trauma course about fires, burns, and victims in enclosed spaces. I remembered how fire and hot gases, once inhaled, could cause swelling in the airways and potentially occlude them. Black sputum and singed faces, like those of the children, were indicators of potential airway compromise. I'd like to think that somehow, I was instrumental in saving their lives, and that they are happy and healthy today, playing with their own children.

That week, two more kids died. They were days apart, but the mechanism of injury was the same—they were falls. They fell because they were standing up in the shopping carts while their mothers were gathering the weeks groceries. Kids' heads are big; the books will say their heads disproportionally large compared with their bodies. When they fall, they almost always land head first and bonk themselves. That was a tough week. I still get a little queasy when I'm in grocery stores and see kids standing in carts. At the risk of sounding too psycho, I always warn their mothers.

I loved that pediatrics ER. The staff was awesome. One clerk was from the state of Georgia. She was a tall, beautiful black woman and her name badge read HNIC. Nurses always like to add letters to their name, but HNIC was something I didn't recognize. So, I asked. She told me, and I just shook my head. Never would I utter the designation that she self-applied, "Head N In Charge!" She was from the South she was "country". Once, she returned from vacation and brought me cotton she picked. We had a huge laugh. She would often proudly go on about how she never needed a man. She would describe how she'd just dim her lights, pour herself a glass of wine, turn on some Barry White with a softly lit candle and then…. She had no need for a man's hot breath all over her. I would just shake my head. Man, I loved her!

Working in that place had meaning. I felt like I was serving a real purpose. We were doing really good work. For years, I stayed with no intention of going anywhere else. One of my co-workers told me that there was no place like it. He could not have been more right.

A 12-month-old came in. She was seizing. I speculated that she got into her mother's cocaine. The child's urine tested positive for the drug, and the doctor asked me how I knew. Who knows how I knew?

As time went on, I was bounced back and forth from the pediatrics ER to the adult ER. By that time, I was an MICN, a Mobile Intensive Care Nurse, which meant I was qualified to answer the paramedic radio. I directed paramedic traffic and made decisions to help medics care for their patients. It was fun, exciting, and I learned a whole lot more! The alarm would go off and the MICNs would run to the radio. Everyone wanted to take the calls!

Being an MICN required continued education, so we attended lectures and reviewed interesting calls. Sometimes, your call was reviewed, which could cause you to squirm in your seat. Still, we were always reassured that the purpose was never punitive, but to enhance everyone's knowledge. It never was punitive, until…

CHAPTER 8

MICN TAPE REVIEW

A new nurse took the position of prehospital care coordinator and hired her girlfriend as an assistant. It didn't really matter much to me, but it was odd how they became so serious, so important, and so mean over the course of a single day.

A new MICN took a call. The patient was unresponsive with a very slow heartbeat, so the MICN ordered atropine, a drug that increased the patient's heart rate. Well, the patient arrived at the ER alive, but soon died. He had a big bleed in his head—a hemorrhagic stroke—which there was no way to see that from our seats in the ER. The MICN was sternly reprimanded and was told he had killed the patient by elevating the heart rate. That nurse never answered a call again and left the ER soon after.

I watched the behavior of these two women with disgust. They came after me over a call. Goose stepping into the ER, they were furious, and said I'd ordered the wrong medication for a patient. I told them to listen to the tape. The patient did not get the medication. As the patient's heart rhythm changed, the medic was directed to hold the medication that I had initially ordered. It wasn't given. They wouldn't listen to me. Instead, they were ready to fry me. We went to their office, where we sat and listened to the tape. The sequence unfolded exactly as I described, and the medication was held. I never received an apology and needless to say never thought much of those two thereafter. That same feeling of being punished for something always found its way back to me.

During a tape review, we were discussing if and when a patient could decide not to be transferred to the hospital. In question was a case where a man passed out on the toilet and his wife called 911.When medics arrived, he was awake and refused the transfer. As we discussed the case, I raised my hand and posed another question (I wanted to stick a bug up the coordinator's…). I asked if we could order the medics to wipe the patient's butt, so he wouldn't arrive soiled in the ER. She kicked me out of the review. I couldn't stop laughing.

Another time, I was at a review and they would play a game like *Jeopardy*. When we gave correct answers, we accumulated points. I always loved winning (and still do). The final challenge was to identify the 12 cranial nerves. I answered without hesitation. I learned an acronym in school: On Old Olympus' Towering Tops, A Finn And German Viewed Some Hops. I asked if I could share another acronym I had learned, to which she said, "Please do!" It went as follows: OOO, To Touch And Feel A Girl's Vagina, Ah Heaven! She kicked me out of the class again. I won the game and had an even greater laugh!

Soon, there were plenty of MICNs and I didn't really feel the rush to answer the calls. The coordinator and her assistant took the fun away.

CHAPTER 9

BEING IN CHARGE AND SEX IN THE ER

Being in charge of the adult ER was a very interesting experience. I took the job seriously. I would go out to triage waiting room and bring patients back, help with the flow of the department and admissions, and facilitate communications with the senior resident. Between all these tasks, there was never a dull moment.

I felt that some of the staff resented the fact that I was in charge. Perhaps they wanted to be in charge, or simply didn't like being directed by me. There were always attitudes everywhere. At times, I had to remember I was a man in a female-dominated profession. Perhaps some of the women resented a man in charge, I don't know. Honestly, it was easier for me to have my own patient assignment. Either way, I did my job the best I could.

I asked a tech to bring a patient up to the obstetrics floor the woman had been transferred to us in pre-term labor. The ER tech refused, so I took the patient up. Consequently, I had to leave the department I was in charge of because the tech would not do her job! Go figure! The technicians served little purpose in the ER. For example, the technician on the day shift was rarely around. When he was present, he was drunk. He spent his shifts drinking Seagram's V.O., and cornering the young female ER nurses attempting to steal kisses. What's worse, he got to retire with a pension! The technicians on the PM shift weren't much better; it was like they were always doing you a favor when you asked them to do their job. I always thought that was a bit of a joke. The techs in the pediatrics ER were incredible, however. They worked hard, knew their jobs, and did it. They were always a pleasure to work beside.

I encountered other crazy obstacles at times, particularly as I tried to run that adult side. There were times I could not locate the storeroom keys. I needed supplies and there was no way to get them. Yeah, it was a bit frustrating. Invariably the keys only showed up at the end of the shift. When I did finally get into storeroom, I would find pairs of panties on the floor! One had to wonder who was taking care of the patients during these orgies. Other times I would order an EKG STAT and the EKG technician would never show. Rumor had it she was banging doctors two at a time upstairs in the EKG lab! All I could say was, are you kidding me?

One day, a trauma was about to arrive. I alerted the trauma team but could not locate the senior ER resident. I was looking all over for him because he was the doctor who would be running the trauma case. Finally, the doctor appeared. He looked wiped out, spent, and was a bit clammy, too. I asked him what the heck was going on and informed him we had a trauma about to knock on the door. He confessed he was in the back getting a blow job in the eye room from one of the nurses! Again, are you kidding me? It was a wonder how the place ran at all.

Now, the eye room had an instrument called a slit lamp it used for eye exams. It would emit an ultraviolet light that would help in identifying abrasions on the cornea. I walked into the eye room once to find an orthopedic resident with two interns taking hits off the blue tank. They were all getting high on the nitrous oxide, the laughing gas. The purple light was on, illuminating the dark room and they looked like they should have been listening to some Hendrix, some "Purple Haze" it was psychedelic!

I took a couple breaths from the tank myself and walked out of the room. Down the hall, I could see the attending physician with a police officer coming my way. I asked where they were going, and he told me they needed the eye room, the officer had something in his eye. I asked the doctor to give me a minute to clean up the room he responded, "No, that's okay." Looking the doctor straight in the eye—this guy was a very serious man—I told him I really needed to clean the room. He stared at me, I stared back at him. He knew something was up and gave me the nod they then rerouted back into the ER.

As they turned around, I went running right back into the eye room and told those doctors that the attending was on his way in. They scattered like cockroaches in the light! I'd like to think that somehow, I was instrumental in saving their careers and made a difference in their lifelong practice in orthopedic medicine. Just maybe thousands of people may have new hips and knees today, because of my rapid nursing intervention.

One of the things that I liked about being in charge was that I was in a great position to help the nursing staff with patient care when there was a need.

Rounds were a time when all the interns and residents would meet with the attending physician. During that hour, many ER cases would be presented, and discussed thoroughly, those present would receive a deeper education, the patient care would be directed. Rounds were scheduled at eight in the morning and eight in the evening. It was nice because the staff nurses would get a bit of a break until rounds were over, at which point new orders would come out flying, there would be a renewed flurry of activity.

One particular evening during rounds, I was freed up and asked a nurse if she needed help. She said, "No, but Bill looked like he could use some." I went over to Bill and he looked like he was ready to cry. An ER resident was with him. It was as if they'd lost their best friend. I asked what was going on. Bill told me his patient was dead. I listened as he told me that he gave the patient a sandwich, visited another patient on the other side of the curtain and upon returning to the first patient, found him dead. I saw the patient in question. His eyes were closed, he was sitting upright with a juice box in his hand. I truly believed Bill was messing with me because the situation didn't make any sense. Bill was a great nurse and the doctor with him had a lot of experience. I shook the patient and he did not respond. I checked his carotid artery for a pulse, and after realizing it was absent I asked Bill and the doctor if they wanted to start CPR. I guess it was the jolt they needed. We began resuscitation. They were right, the man was dead.

Other obstacles presented themselves, too. I found that if a patient was to be admitted to the coronary care unit, the nurses up there would almost always say they'd call when the bed was ready. I, however, learned to go up to the sixth floor, walk into the unit, and check for myself. More often than not, the bed was clean and ready for the admission. I would then ask if I could bring the patient up. Obviously, I didn't make too many friends up there.

Another nice thing about being in charge was that I was always working beside the clerks. These guys knew me from nursing school days and they saw me grow up in that ER.

We always had fun and shared a bunch of laughs retelling old stories. I always had a sense of gratification by the end of the shift. As busy and crazy as things got, we all survived. We were a team.

CHAPTER 10

DRIVEN TO TEARS

I didn't often tear up on the job. ER nursing requires a lot of strength. I personally found I had to somehow get to a place where I would not be affected by the events, not emotionally, and certainly not at work. Over time, it proved possible to weaken.

I was working in the pediatrics ER and a police officer showed up with two young boys. The kids looked fine. There was no sign of illness or injury that I could see. I asked the officer what 's going on, why are you here? He looked straight at me and told me the kids were sexually assaulted by their father. I had to take a deep breath. There was a searing pain inside me. Not only could I not fathom such an act, but I was also broken as I thought about how these two brothers, these two beautiful young boys could go on after what their father had done to them.

Another boy arrived, and I was to care for him. He was another victim of child abuse. He was about 10 years old and as cute as could be. I had to assess him and document the purple and yellow bruising, representative of different stages of healing. I charted the lacerations on his genitals, the cigarette burns over his body, and the torn skin around his anus. This young boy was so sweet. He had these big brown eyes—my eyes began to leak. I could not help crying as I charted what I saw, everywhere I looked there was more evidence. All I wanted to do was to bring him into my home, love him, and give him a good life. He was medically cleared from the ER and was taken away by Child Services. I still see his face today.

Things add up after a while. I was working back at the adult side. As I was starting an IV on a patient, the double doors of the ER opened, and I could see a young girl enter. She was blond and looked like a beach girl. She ran into our trauma room and all I heard were nonstop cries. They were pleas. She was begging and pleading, "Daddy wake up, wake up daddy please, daddy don't be dead, please daddy!" Wiping tears from my eyes, I taped the IV down, wondering how much more of this I could possibly take. Sometimes reality gets to be too much. I flashed back to the day I saw my own dad taken away. I knew what she'd be in for. I began to wonder, who does this for a living?

As if these experiences weren't enough, they never stopped. Only once did I walk out of the ER. The patient was a 15-year-old girl from Central America. She was beautiful, but she was dead. The story went that she was a teenage prostitute who had overdosed. We worked on this young girl, but all the resuscitative efforts were pointless. Her life was gone, over. I was overcome with a deep sadness for her. I walked out of the building and cried by the ambulance entrance. One of my co-workers came out and asked if I was okay. I said yeah, wiped my tears, and walked back in. We had more patients.

The next day, I was walking into work and a nurse told me I'd just missed it. I asked her what I missed. She said a patient opened a window in his room upstairs, jumped out, and died by the ambulance entrance. Missed it? I was glad I missed it. Who would want to see that? Then I realized I was just there last night crying over the young girl who died from the drug overdose. I guess the hits just keep coming.

We got a call. A young girl and her mother were run over in a crosswalk by a drunk driver. The paramedics were frantic. We got the kid, a beautiful girl who was on her way home from a piano recital. She was hit hard; it looked like every bone in her body was broken and her eyes were purple and swollen shut. I started two IVs, and she was intubated. We were pushing O negative blood. Her heart slowed, then stopped. CPR could not save her. Her mother made it into surgery. She survived but lost both her legs, oh yeah, her daughter too.

As much as I loved what I was doing and where I was working, I was beginning to think that perhaps it was time for a change.

CHAPTER 11

ANOTHER MANAGER

Managing the emergency department did not carry much longevity. You could say the manager's office could have used a revolving door, given the frequency with which the position was vacated.

Most of the managers we had were pretty clueless. I recall one manager observing me as I drew up some medication. She was convinced I was making an error. The medication was in a concentration of five milligrams per milliliter, she wanted one milligram. So, I pulled the syringe and drew up 0.2 milliliters of volume. Now the manager was having a fit. I had to show her the multiplication three times, and she still couldn't get it: 5 x 0.2=1. I couldn't help but wonder how she got the job.

We did get a new manager, and she didn't have a very good vibe. She never really had much to say and rarely made any eye contact. It was obvious that she was gay. I gathered she had no appreciation for the men in the department. Her girlfriend was always present in her office. I thought that was a bit odd being that girlfriend was not an employee, but I knew I'd be better off keeping my distance and try my best to stay under her radar.

One day, she was talking to one of the male nurses. Jack was a good nurse who worked the night shift. I didn't know what the conversation was about, but I heard the manager tell him that he could not say the word fuck! He just looked at her and walked away. All I heard him saying was, "Fuck, fuck, fuck, fuck, fuck!" I had a great laugh. Jack lost his job.

A few more of the guys on nights were gone shortly thereafter. It came as a surprise to me. When I got back to the adult side after a few shifts in the pediatrics ER, I came to find my buddies no longer worked there. For one reason or another, they were all let go.

One day, I was called into the manager's office, but was not informed as to why. I was surprised to see the director of nursing there. Her name was Cynthia. Now, Cynthia and I always had a good relationship. She hired me as a new nurse and gave me the ER job I always wanted. At one point, I was going to transfer out to the coronary care unit. She came down to the ER and asked me to stay. I knew that's what she wanted and that it would be better for me to comply. As a result, I ended up staying for another 10 years.

During our meeting, the manager informed me that I could no longer have the schedule I have had for years, since I had started in the place. She said it was hurting the department. I went on to argue that point and also gave reasons why the schedule worked for me and how it in fact benefitted the department. My needs basically revolved around babysitting. She displayed no concern over me or my family's needs and was obviously intent on disrupting my schedule.

I sat back in my chair and said I can't help feeling a bit discriminated against. At this, she exploded, and I knew I had her! I looked straight at Cynthia, then turned to the manager and said, "You know, since you've come on board here I've noticed that I am the only straight white male left in the department! Rich and Tony are gay Filipino men, Thomas is black, and all the other straight white male nurses are gone. Now you want to mess with my schedule!

Cynthia knew I was onto something. Immediately, the meeting was over. My schedule never changed, and I never had too much to do with that manager. She didn't last much longer.

CHAPTER 12

TRYING TO STAY AFLOAT

The more you do something, the better you become. Nursing is no exception. You become better at starting IVs, your assessment skills get sharper, and in time you can anticipate patients' needs and doctors' orders. It's experience that makes ER nursing easier, and it takes time there is no shortcut. For the same reason, being new is overwhelming. If you're fortunate, you'll work with a good crew that never leaves you drowning.

I was lucky enough to be surrounded by a number of excellent nurses. When I was still new, I had a patient to whom I was giving blood. She also needed an IV infusion of medicine for her seizure disorder. The IVs blew, and I was sunk. I couldn't do anything for the patient. I asked another nurse to find a vein. She successfully stuck the patient, and I was back in business. Helplessness is not a pleasant feeling to have as an ER nurse because you always want to do the best you can for your patient. It sucks when your best isn't good enough.

Years later, the department acquired a rapid fluid infuser that could deliver almost 700 milliliters of warm fluid a minute! No one would bleed out when this thing was hooked up!

I was working in the pediatrics ER when I was asked to help a new nurse on the adult side. I walked over there and could see the fear in her eyes. Her patient was vomiting all kinds of blood and the doctors were scoping his stomach right there. It was a big mess. The patient needed blood immediately. She had the rapid infuser but didn't know its operation. Well, Thomas and I jumped on the thing! We were slamming the blood into the patient, starting more lines, and joking and laughing the whole time. These out-of-control emergencies were the kind of thing we lived for. We had a blast, and the patient did well.

The next day, the new nurse found me again in the pediatrics ER. She said, "Thank you so much for yesterday. If it wasn't for you, I would have never come back!" I recalled when I was new, standing scared next to the supply cart. I remembered the troubles I had inserting IVs. In response to her comment, I told her I was happy to help anytime she ever needed it. I imagine she grew to be an incredible ER nurse because she had that quality.

CHAPTER 13

SOCIETAL ILLS

During my time in this particular ER, I saw a lot of things change, some not necessarily for the better.

The changes in medicine were marvelous. Drugs were developed that could open coronary arteries and save people from deadly heart attacks. Other medicines showed up that could control chaotic heart arrhythmias. Studies were conducted that shaped pediatric airway management. Despite all these wonderful advances in emergency medicine, the society we worked to help seemed to be moving in the opposite direction.

I saw kids coming into the ER victims of drive-by shootings. Suicides were occurring more frequently, even on the beach! Stores were robbed in the neighborhood. A lady fell and broke her hip while getting her purse snatched. The kids who robbed her were sent up for murder since the lady died in the operating room. Other gunshot victims were transferred in from a movie theatre where they were waiting to see a movie about a gang of female bank robbers. Two of the nurses I worked with were carjacked in the hospital parking lot.

Our triage booth had now become encased in bulletproof glass. We would buzz one person in at a time. All the while, we were guarded by an armed police officer. Metal detectors were installed at every entrance, and hundreds of weapons were confiscated. If we called security, they would show up with leather gloves on their fists and proceed to beat the patient into submission. Five nurses I worked with carried handguns in their fanny packs, where bandages and tape used to fill their front pocket. That pocket now could be torn away to pull out a handgun and extra clips. It was crazy. I understood it, everything was out of control.

Security was called on a patient who was acting out. Two officers showed up and began to pummel him. The ER doctor was yelling, "Take it easy, we don't want to make him a trauma patient!" I told him to shut up and let them do their job, so he could do his. The last thing I ever wanted was to call these guys and have them not show up! We would then be in a world of hurt for sure!

The paramedic radio went off, it was a stab wound victim who had been riding his bike. Some guys just got out of their car and stabbed him in the stomach while they were at a stop light just to steal his bicycle. Later, two high school kids were carjacked. They were shot in the head and killed. Their car was found just a mile down the road from where they were jacked. Turns out they were exchange students, spending a year in America. They returned to their home, reunited with their families dead. I was really beginning to think perhaps now would be a good time for a change. Another kid showed up in the pediatrics ER, a victim of a drive-by shooting. I found out it was at the park where I bring my kids to play on the tire swing. I knew it was time to go.

I'd made some good friends over the years. Somehow, they'd all moved to the same area. It was outside of the city, a small town bordered with beautiful country roads. We visited, and I thought it would be a great place to raise the family. I could be back working with my old buddies, in an environment that was safe and sane. Certainly, the opportunity was something to really think about.

I wasn't sure, though. I loved the hospital I worked in, the pediatrics ER, and the adult side. My aspiration was to become an ER nurse, and somehow, I considered this place my home. I loved the action, the doctors were awesome, we were always learning, plus I knew everyone. I was familiar with the location of everything on each of the 10 floors. I would recall my experiences working for the registry, in the private sector and what that was like. All the while, I could hear my old buddy tell me that there was no place like this place. I remained uncertain.

CHAPTER 14

PUMPING STOMACHS

Back in the day, patients who presented with drug overdoses would get their stomachs pumped. That meant a tube, much like a garden hose, had to be placed into their stomach. If the patient was conscious, it was often a bit of a struggle. We would have to tie their hands down to get it done. If the patient fought too hard, we could also place a piece of plastic in their mouth to keep it open while slipping the hose in. If that didn't work, there was always the nose, you know that hurt!

The procedure certainly had risks. The patient could vomit, and the contents could end up in their lungs. We had to be very careful. The placement was always confirmed, either by the return of gastric contents or by injection of air into the tube while listening for bubbles in the stomach.

After pumping the stomach until what returned was clear, we would administer charcoal to absorb whatever was left in the digestive tract. Charcoal was thick and gritty. If spilled, it would leave an indelible stain. I chuckled every time the charcoal exploded from pushing it too hard into the tube during its administration. A black shower would spray all over the doctor's white lab coat. Oh, they'd be pissed! It was never coming out!

At times I would get to work with this one doctor. He was very smart and appeared to be always in command of the department. A kid came into the trauma bed unresponsive. We assumed a drug overdose was the cause. In no time at all, the patient was intubated to protect his airway and then placed on a ventilator. I dropped an Ewald tube (the name of the hose) to pump his stomach. I was blown away by what came out. He filled the two-liter bag with what appeared to be a gut full of whiskey. It was like it came right out of the bottle, the smell was so strong. We could have started pouring drinks! That doctor saved the kid's life! The man was an animal and a blast to work with!

One thing I always found a bit ironic was the administration of medications called tricyclic antidepressants. Turns out that this class of drug can be very lethal. It is used to combat depression, so how was it that the most dangerous drugs are prescribed to those suffering from depression and possibly more likely to commit suicide?

I had a patient who had a tricyclic overdose. I placed her on a cardiac monitor, prepared the Ewald tube, and explained the procedure to the patient. Two residents and their interns were at the bedside to observe the procedure. I started placing the tube, when the attending physician walked into the room. I recall what he once said about nobody caring. As he approached, he told the group of doctors assembled around the gurney that I was born for this ER and that there were not too many people you could say that about. I thanked him for the compliment.

I then proceeded to place the hose into the patient's mouth. She grabbed it from me and said, "Just give it to me." She began to swallow the tube herself, shoving it down her own throat. I never

ever saw anything like that before. I was awestruck. I couldn't help myself, and without any delay, right there and then, I asked her to marry me! The group of doctors around the bed lost it. They were all crying with laughter, tears streaming down their faces. Shame on me!

Another patient arrived, accompanied by police. He had ingested all the cocaine he was dealing, so as not to get arrested for the possession. As they walked over to me, the kid fell unconscious on the floor. We got him on the gurney. He was pulseless, and the cardiac monitor revealed ventricular tachycardia. He suffered a lethal heart arrhythmia and died. Again, I placed a tag on his toe, zipped him up into the plastic bag, and sent him up to be refrigerated.

CHAPTER 15

SCALES

Scales are often used in medicine. A standardization of measurement can be used to grasp relative proportions. Some scales are used to measure weight, while others can be used to grade, and still others can measure an amount or distance and even pressures. When I say that we use a scale to measure weight, I don't necessarily mean the patient's weight. When I was drawing blood on the neonatal babies, I would weigh their wet diapers. One gram of weight in a soaked diaper equaled one milliliter of urine, which was an easy way to measure the baby's urine output.

Other scales were used in a variety of patient assessments. We used a scale to measure a hematocrit (the patient's percentage of red blood cells in their circulating blood volume). A tube of blood would be spun down in a centrifuge, placed against a scale, and from it that value of could be derived.

Some scales were used to measure pressures in the body. Invasive lines in the chest, heart, or head could be set up to yield certain values. The scales could be calibrated against centimeters of water or millimeters of mercury. There are all kinds of ways to measure stuff.

Turns out, there are two scales to measure a woman's beauty in the ER. Sometimes, an attractive nurse would walk by. Other times, new female interns arrived in the department. It wasn't uncommon for them to be graded on a scale from one to ten. I remember when one particularly attractive new staff member arrived while I was talking with the attending physician, Dr. Kirk. I found him to be a most fascinating man with a long resume. He'd had spent many years doing research that not only drove emergency cardiac care, but also saved lives and shaped treatment protocols all over the country. He was and still is one of the most brilliant individuals I've ever known.

As this young lady passed us by, I looked over at Dr. Kirk and made mention that by all means I felt she was a ten! Everything about her was perfect, jaw-dropping beauty. Now, Dr. Kirk looked over at me and said, "No, she's about a four."

"Are you kidding me?" I was wondering what planet he was on.

His reply was that the lady was a four on the Kirk scale!

The Kirk scale? What is that? This guy spent years in learning institutions and many years after that in research. He was well published. I could only guess he knew about something I did not. Perhaps this scale was of his own invention, which I was to learn it most certainly was. He told me the Kirk scale was based on how many Clydesdales it would take to drag the young lady off his face! Turns out that on the Kirk scale, four is good, very good!

CHAPTER 16

ALL TIED DOWN

When I went back to work in the pediatrics ER, one of my buddies came up to me and said, "Man, you missed it yesterday." I asked him to clarify. He told me an eight-year-old boy was admitted after being shot in the face by his father. Turns out the dad had to tell the kid to go back to bed and after the third time, just shot him. He arrived still in his Batman pajamas. Somehow, I'm glad I did miss it.

The next day, I was working in the adult side. We were in the middle of summer and it was hot. Now, the local police department had squad cars that were black with white doors.

They brought in a man under arrest. The man looked like he was in a lot of pain from the second and third degree burns all over his chest and abdomen. He looked like he was cooked. I guess while placing him under arrest, they slammed him down on the hood of the cruiser. The man was shirtless, so when they lifted him off the car his skin of his chest was seared by the hood.

One of the duties as charge nurse was stocking a stainless-steel medicine cabinet in the middle of the ER. One thing I noticed was that whenever the State was coming, doors would appear miraculously on the cabinet that could be locked. Whenever the State would leave, the doors would somehow disappear. Anyway, as I was stocking the shelves another law enforcement agency brought in someone they had apprehended. He entered hog-tied on a gurney. He was face down with his legs and arms all tied together. I greeted the officers and asked what was up with the guy. They told me he was on PCP. Now I've seen a lot of people whacked out on PCP. They are always completely out of control. It takes a lot of manpower and medication to knock them down. However, this guy was completely still. I asked them if he was breathing, and they said yes. The ER tech was walking by the patient. I said, "Hey Steve, see if that guy has a pulse."

He checked and said, "Yeah, he's got a pulse." I kept stocking as I tried to figure where I could place our new patient. All the while, I was looking at him. He wasn't moving. I stopped what I was doing and checked his carotid artery to find that he was pulseless and not breathing! The officers quickly cut the zip ties that secured him. We got him to a bed and began CPR. All resuscitative efforts were futile. He was dead. I tagged him, bagged him, and up to the refrigerator he went.

The paramedic radio was alarming about another cardiac arrest. He was a middle-aged man who arrived intubated by the paramedics. We took over CPR, gave him a couple rounds of epinephrine, and shocked him. It was too late, he died. Moments later, his wife arrived with two children, obviously in a state of disbelief. She asked, "Where was he found?" It was reported to her that the 911 call came from home. She said but he wasn't home. Quickly, it was deduced the man was at the other woman's home. That had to be really hard to take. I couldn't imagine her pain. He was gone and that was that.

The nurse who was working the code with me, well, she leaned over and whispered in my ear, "Any man who cheats on his wife deserves to die." I looked at her and thought, "I don't want to be your friend anymore." Where the hell did that come from? Deserves to die?

CHAPTER 17

MAKING FRIENDS AND SPREADING SUNSHINE

The paramedic radio was notifying us that we were to receive a full arrest, another kid. He was a victim of what they called a near drowning. The patient was submerged and unresponsive, but still had vital signs. I guess it wouldn't be near drowning if you died underwater and had no vital signs. Anyway, I was in the pediatrics ER, working with a nurse who prided herself on being published. She had authored chapters for a pediatric emergency book. She was impressed by that and perhaps I should have been, too. I was always a bit annoyed by her because she always attempted to push me around. One day, she walked me into the other ER department (OB-GYN) and asked me to cosign some Demerol she wasted. I looked at her and asked, "You want me to sign for a drug I did not see you pull, on shift I didn't work, in a department I wasn't in?" I just walked away. No way!

A code was arriving. The nurse was frantic and began pushing me to go into the crash room. Obviously, she was out of sorts. I looked at her and asked, "Why do you want me to go in there? Didn't you write the book?" If looks could kill!

I jumped into the crash room. We intubated the patient and immediately began CPR. We gave epinephrine because the patient was in PEA, meaning pulseless electrical activity. It describes a state in which the heart displays electrical energy with a normal conduction pattern but doesn't give a mechanical pulse or muscular contraction. We worked furiously on that child. He did not survive.

On the adult side, one of the nurses was going for her master's degree in nursing. She proudly walked into the department showing off her textbooks. One I could see was a textbook on cardiology. I was never really impressed with her because she was a girl who was always trolling for a doctor. In fact, she was the one crying that day long ago because she was assigned to the pediatrics ER and didn't want to go.

We had ancient cardiac monitors in the ER. Their cables were cracked, and the lead wires were often shot. I was always messing around with them to get them to work. I read a good book on cardiac rhythms and learned how to switch lead wires around to get better waveforms from the old machines. After that, they worked really well for me. The nurse with her cardiology book asked me how I was able to manipulate the monitors. I asked her, "Aren't you the one taking the cardiology classes?" I guess that didn't go over too well either.

Many nurses came and went. Some would burn out in no time and some were there forever. I learned that the ones who lasted the longest often cared the least. It really didn't seem right, but those who were completely careless tended to make it to retirement!

I was walking past a new nurse who carried a nasty attitude. She was one I would generally ignore. She called my name and asked me to look at the IV she was starting because it would not drip the fluid. Well, the IV catheter was in the vein, but it was pointing to his finger. I promptly told her to take it out and turn it around. Man, she was pissed at me! How was I the bad guy? She was the one putting IVs in upside down!

I saw a monitor display a run of ventricular tachycardia (V-tach). It is a cardiac arrhythmia that requires immediate attention. I looked on the assignment board to see which physician was seeing the patient. I called the doctor by his name, as I'd known the doctor for years and I still remembered him when he was a timid medical student. Since he was only 10 feet away from me, I called him by his name again, "Mike, Mike!" He was totally ignoring me. Finally, I called, "Dr. Wilson!"

He walked over to me with an intern who seemed like a nice young lady and said, "Who are you calling Mike, boy!" His left fist was clenched. I guess he was getting ready to swing at me.

I looked at him and replied, "Who are you calling boy, motherfucker!"

I then asked if he was going to hit me. I went to speak with the attending physician who was in charge of the ER, I was pretty jacked up. I grabbed him and said, "I don't know how you're training your boys." I then relayed the details of my interaction with Dr. Wilson. I told the man I'd be happy to take Dr. Wilson outside and beat the shit out of him.

Like a father, he put his arm around me and said, "Now please don't hit the residents."

After 10 plus years in that place, I wasn't making many new friends or spreading much sunshine. It was time to leave. I was getting out of the city! I talked to some of my old friends who assured me I'd get a job. The director of nursing didn't want me to leave. She asked me where I would go, sounding much like a concerned parent. Still, I was confident that the experiences I had gained would land me a nursing job anywhere. It was time to pack.

CHAPTER 18

OPENING NEW DOORS

As luck would have it, I landed a job immediately. I was back in the ER of a small community hospital. I had no idea how small. The director of nursing hired me and gave me a tour. During the tour, she walked me into a room that looked like a regular patient room. It had two gurneys and a little closet with an exam table. She said that this is our emergency room! I was looking everywhere only to realize I was standing in the emergency room. I was dumbfounded. Then a shot of fear ran through me. I realized that the ER I came out of in the city was as large as this entire hospital! This was going to be way different. I knew I had way too much energy for this place.

I had a family to support, so I went to work, and it was killing me. For one 12-hour shift, all I did was take a patient's blood pressure. A couple from the retirement community nearby just walked in and asked if I could check the man's blood pressure. I wasn't sure I could take this kind of pace very much longer.

The place never got busy and the practice of medicine was pretty backwards to say the least. I felt like I'd stepped back in time and had to assume some subservient role. As time went on, I worked in their small ICU and their recovery room also. I made it work largely because I didn't have a choice. The place had a weird vibe. Most of the nurses were stressed and seemed a bit stuck up. This was going to take some getting used to.

One day, the director of nursing asked me to take over management of the ER and ICU. She also wanted me to run the respiratory therapy (RT) department. The position was days full-time and salaried, so I said, "Why not?" I knew nothing of respiratory therapy, but those guys really ran themselves. The ER was basically two beds, and the ICU wasn't going to be too much of a load. There were only six beds and the patients were not that sick.

On my first day as the new manager, I was greeted by one nasty nurse. She walked right up to me and said, "Don't you ever fuck with me!" She approached me two more times that day with the same warning. I had no idea what that was about. The next day, she walked into my office and threw a number of binders down on my desk. She exclaimed she would no longer do the ER schedule. She also resigned from the safety team and the disaster management team. I said okay.

Not sure where to go with her behavior, I decided to speak to the director of nursing. I was beginning to notice that she was not only a raging alcoholic, but also a chain-smoker. Her face was like leather and she appeared anorexic. She was very slow to respond. When she grasped the situation, she said, "Well it seems like that nurse needs to go." I agreed. Well that nurse was never let go, and it was clear to me that my position was one of total accountability without any authority. Months went by and nothing ever changed. I just put my head down and went to work. The rest of the staff was pretty cool, but that nurse was clearly poisonous.

One day, I went up to the director of nurses' office to find a meeting in progress. The nurse who had been giving me grief was accompanied with a union representative, and it appeared they were discussing me. I invited myself in, took a seat, and allowed them to take aim. At one point, I asked if these were formal accusations of harassment. I was ready for the fight. As I stared the nurse and her rep down, they both began to backpedal. I knew the truth, and there were plenty of witnesses. That conversation was done. This wasn't going anywhere.

I was running the ER, ICU, RT, and doing all the Heart Association classes. I was busy. On top of it all, I was reviewing cases and bringing them to committees. At one point, I had to review a case involving the nurse who'd been giving me all that trouble. She was upset that I wasn't supporting her! Now, I was never on a mission to get her and I was willing to go over the chart alongside her.

We looked at the chart and I complemented her on her narrative. The patient was in a third-degree AV block, which means a very slow rhythm that usually requires a pacemaker. She supported her notes with a cardiac rhythm strip, which was great. In the medication column, she charted she gave 100 milligrams of lidocaine, which was used to abolish ventricular beats. Now, the problem is that the patient's ventricles were the only pacemaker firing to contract the heart muscle. She charted in her narrative that the patient then flatlined and supported that with a flatline rhythm strip. I responded that she gave the wrong drug for the wrong rhythm. The patient died. How was I to support that? Her response was, "The doctor ordered it."

Soon afterwards, I reviewed another chart. Here, the patient received tissue plasminogen activator (tPA), a treatment designed to dissolve blood clots in the coronary artery. The clots were obstructing flow and causing a heart attack. The chart stated the patient's blood pressure spiked, his pupil blew, and he stopped breathing indicating a bleed in his head. That was it! I could not figure this one out! I asked, "Well, did you ventilate the patient? Was he intubated? Did you call neurology?" All the responses were negative! I then asked, "You all just sat there and watched him die?"

Her response was, "The other nurse said she had seen this before stating it doesn't go well." I was left with the impression they did nothing but stand by and watch until the patient expired!

I was also working at a couple of the other hospitals in the community. The one where all my old friends worked was asking me to join full time. I thought that would mean more money, less hours and less BS!

At the time, I was pulling some shifts in another ER where I worked per diem. It was like a little county hospital. It seemed nice enough, but like anything, time would tell. One Sunday, I was working in their critical area, which had four beds. The radio went off. We were getting a patient. The other nurse on duty was reading the paper when the patient arrived. I met the medics, got the patient in the bed, and went to work. Soon, the radio went off again. I was given the next patient by the charge nurse as the other nurse on duty kept reading the paper and made no effort to help. A third patient arrived and was directed to the critical area. I was again assigned that patient while the other nurse remained sitting on the counter by the nurse's station continuing her read of the Sunday funnies. I asked the charge nurse what was going on. He just shook his head. It was obvious that he was not about to resolve the issue. I had three patients while she had none. I thought it was crazy. I did another shift in that ER and was getting the feeling that things weren't quite right. It became obvious that none of the staff really cared for the manager. In time, I would understand why.

A young girl about four years old was admitted. She had been bitten by a dog and suffered a number of lacerations and avulsions to her face. The parents and child were pretty traumatized, as you could imagine. I wanted to do my best to console them and take care of their baby.

A nurse walked over with a paramedic student and said that she wanted him to start the IV on the young girl. I spoke with her and expressed that I did not think it was a good time. The girl and the parents had been through a lot, so I asked that the student practice on someone else. She was the charge nurse and her arrogance overrode any compassion she may have had. They stuck the patient twice and failed. I overheard her tell the doctor that they couldn't get the IV and were calling the IV team. Without saying anything, I went back to my patient, placed the IV, gave the Versed and fentanyl to sedate her, and told the doctor she was ready to get stitched up. The charge nurse became irate with me. I didn't care, I cared for my patient. I had years of pediatrics ER experience and began to think the nurses here really sucked. Needless to say, I made another enemy.

During the same shift, I was asked to bring a patient to the surgery department. The receiving nurse was sitting at her desk. As I attempted to give my report, she never got up, turned, or made any effort to listen to me. I repeated that I wanted to give my report, but she was having none of it. The anesthesiologist and orthopedic surgeon arrived. I gave them the report and handed them the chart, returning to my department. As I walked, I was thinking, "This place is just insane." But I was in for more.

As I returned to the department, the paramedic radio alarmed to tell us we were getting a patient who was unresponsive. It turned out that the patient fell in the bathtub. Not only was she unresponsive, but she also had a very rapid heart rate. The decision was to intubate the patient and begin an IV infusion of procainamide to control her heart rate. Once she was stable, I accompanied her to the CT scan. Upon return to the ER, she was evaluated by the admitting physician. I called to report to the ICU, and the nurse told me to bring her in five minutes.

I prepared the patient for the transfer, and we brought her up to the ICU. The respiratory therapist brought in the ventilator, so I bagged the patient for another minute before she was placed on the bed and the vent. Upon my return to the ER, my manager called me. She screamed so loud, I turned the phone from my ear. The doctor and I were rolling our eyes. The manager was accusing me of bringing a patient to the ICU without giving report or knowing anything about the patient, and then transferring her without a bed having been prepared. I retorted, "I accepted the patient from the medics, started the IVs and gave all the meds. I've been with her in CT scan, and gave report to the nurse who told me to come up in five minutes." Obviously, this manager was insane!

I saw her pull a shift in the ER once. She was screaming at a patient, belittling him. She reminded me of nurse Dale who screamed at that most pleasant old man way back when. She was pathetic, and I had no respect for her. Soon after this transpired, I was called into her office. She began to reprimand me for bringing a patient to surgery without giving report to anyone. If I was drinking milk, it would have come out my nose. I was not about to be intimidated, so I asked her, "Do you really think I would do such a thing?" I told her that her friend Cary refused to take the report, never got off her seat, and proceeded to ignore me completely. As a result, I had to speak directly to the patient's doctors. I told her she couldn't be more wrong! I didn't blink!

The staff was required to attend a trauma class. I knew trauma pretty well after 10 years in a trauma center. Even so, I paid a lot of attention to the class material. As the class concluded, there was a written exam, followed by a clinical evaluation. I whipped through the test. I was the first one done! In the back of the room, there were a number of other testing stations. I demonstrated all the intervention skills and was having a ball with the instructor. She appreciated my energy and skill; we had some good laughs. My manager was also in the class. She had yet to finish the written exam. She turned around to see me flying through the testing effortlessly and scoffed at me. I remember thinking, "What a sorry woman." Rather than celebrating that she hired a competent, skilled, and knowledgeable nurse, she could only show disdain. It was then that I really understood why the rest of her staff harbored such a dislike towards her. Sad, pathetic really.

Now, the hospital where some of my old friends worked, had more shifts opening up. A position became available and I applied. They got me in. Giving up the management job and switching basically meant more money and less hours at work. In short, it was a no-brainer! I made the switch and left the management job. After my departure, they hired three people to do the job that I was doing on my own. Funny how that happened!

As I walked into the ER, I saw an old friend of mine Dr Vas. He was a doctor I knew from the county days. He was really happy to see me. He started shouting that I was the best nurse he ever worked with and expressed how glad he was that I was here. It was great seeing him again! Yet only a few minutes later, he approached me and said that two of the nurses asked him, "What makes him so good? You never say that to us!" I was shocked! These were 40-year-old women. Who would behave like that? I also came to realize that the community was very small. Everyone knew everyone else. The other places where I'd done some shifts had nurses who knew these nurses from way back. It was one big clique, and they all talked.

I was delighted that I was in this new job alongside some old friends. It was here I would spend the rest of my nursing career. I was stable, or so I thought!

CHAPTER 19

FRIENDS AND FOES

When I look back at the time I spent in that ER, I think it is fair to say that I have never been around a more pathological group of people in my life. Without exaggeration, almost everyone talked shit about each other. It was as if they all harbored some kind of resentment towards one another for what reasons I would never know. Collectively, almost all of them had one thing in common: they hated patients.

Now, to be fair a few of the doctors were really good. Dr. Vas was sharp and quick. Though it was always a challenge to keep up with him, it was a pleasure and a relief to work beside him, he was good, he was a friend. Dr. Hope was my favorite. She was brilliant, skilled, and there was no BS ever. I knew her from back in the county days. I remember I saw her once with a syringe held in her mouth gripped in her teeth while she was ripping out a patient's ingrown toenail with a pair of pliers. She was awesome, she was an animal! I could work with her the rest of my days in perfect unison. I'm not sure how much she was appreciated by some of her colleagues, but they were a bunch of losers anyway. She was better than them. She outshined them she ran circles around them. Since then, we have remained lifelong friends.

One thing I appreciated most about her was that I could say, "Hey, can you look at this patient?" and she would! One time, this kid was pretty sick. I called her in and in no time, she called out for fluids, labs, blood cultures, a blood gas, and antibiotics. The patient was blown away, he didn't get her intention, and as the doctor left he started saying she was kind of a bitch. I responded that was hardly the case, and in fact she was exactly the doctor he wanted caring for him. She's the kind of doctor anyone would be lucky to get, she came to work and saved lives.

It's kind of funny that her name was Hope, that's just what she would give you!

One doctor regularly left the department to work out and couldn't be found for hours he was at the gym while his patients were in a gurney. Another rarely saw any patients and always dragged his feet. Still another doctor would fall asleep at his computer, drooling all over his shirt; the man was a joke a truly disgusting sight to look at. There was a doctor who seemed completely miserable with a permanent scowl plastered on his face. Evidently, he was going through a divorce. I remember him being mean to just about everyone. One day, he got right up into my face. I don't know what had set him off; he wouldn't budge. I finally asked him if he was going to ask me to dance! I just shook my head. Another doctor would go on and on about her brilliance. She graduated from a prestigious medical school and believed she was way above the rest, smarter than all of her colleagues. Her name was Dr. Drew. More about her later. This place was certainly a cast of characters; it should have had clowns and elephants all enclosed in a Big Top!

Most of the nurses were all friends with each other. Some had spouses working in the department as well. As I said, it was a small community. Everyone knew everyone. They were all big fishes in a very small pond, and I was the new guy! The truth is, they were neither very skilled nor experienced in the ER.

I watched them pick on one particular nurse for quite some time. I liked the nurse and found her to be a very kind person and very caring. After some time, the whole gang was successful in getting her fired. I remember thinking it wouldn't be long before they came after me. Well, it didn't take long.

One day, I was working and a friend of mine brought in one of his kids. He fell and fractured his patella, so he was in a lot of pain. I informed the physician and pulled up some Demerol to give for the pain. I was about to inject it when the charge nurse told me to go to lunch. I responded, "Would you just give me a minute and let me give this medication?" The charge nurse and her husband both demanded I not give the medication and go to lunch. I injected the medication I had drawn up into my patient's leg. In doing so, I made some enemies for life!

At times, I was invited to party with the crew after work. They went to each other's homes, got high, drank, and jumped in the hot tub together. I always declined. For one, I wasn't interested in partying with them. Even more importantly, though, I wanted to get home to my family. One of the nurses, she was a real flirt, had asked me to come into the nursing lounge for a second. I followed her in, and as the door closed she dropped her scrub pants to show me the white lace panties she was wearing. I realized I'd better leave before I got in some kind of trouble. I was afraid of possibly having to defend myself against some sexual assault charges or whatever else could come down.

One day, when I was in the triage booth, the same nurse came in to sit beside me and opened up a sex toy catalogue. She began showing me her preferred toys, she told me she liked a lot of power! The doctor that would drool all over himself arrived and paged through the book also. Then, the ER clerk came in and was voicing which toy she would like to use on me! I was wondering who was taking care of the all the patients. These guys were whacked, I had to get up and leave. After all, I wanted to keep my job. Yet another nurse came by to tell me she was wearing her boyfriend's underwear. They'd just had sex in the parking lot during her lunch break, her boyfriend was one of the intensive care doctors. The place was crazy. How crazy? At one point, they both came into the ER overdosed!

As if this wasn't enough, we had one staff nurse that was also a nursing instructor. She taught students at the local junior college, her name was Milly. One day my jaw dropped as I witnessed Milly grab the rectal thermometer and place it under her patients' tongue. Yeah that's right she took the red probe and put it into her patients' mouth.

I triaged a patient who had a high fever and an elevated heart rate of 140. She was sick. I notified Dr. Hope as I put her in a bed. I looked around for the charge nurse, but he was nowhere to be found. As a result, I began to work the patient up. As I was about to insert the IV, the charge nurse arrived and ordered me not to start the IV. I was right there, it would have taken me a second. The woman was the sickest patient in the ER by far. Well, I ignored him, started the IV, and got the blood. He was pissed and called the nursing supervisor.

I was in a state of disbelief. I was being counseled for taking care of a very ill patient. I told the guy that he'd never direct my nursing care. He then shot up out his chair, I assume to attack me. I stood up out of my chair as the nursing supervisor jumped in between us. I found myself in administration the very next day. I had to recite the blow-by-blow of events. It was ridiculous. In my mind, this guy should have gotten the axe. As it was, he had stated that he was now afraid to work with me. I laughed, remembering how he jumped up to attack me! He was also about six inches taller and had me by about 100 pounds. Eventually, he was terminated for fondling a patient's genitals. I knew there was something very wrong about that guy.

Time went by and I made a point of going to work, doing my job the best I could, and going home. Even so, the place kept getting crazier. The nurses really didn't care about much of anything or anyone. The ER had 18 beds, and we were staffed with five nurses. The rack was full of charts for patients waiting to be seen. I watched these guys walk by the rack as though it were invisible. At times, I took up to eight patients. It was crazy. The other nurses just didn't care.

I was working my tail off and saw that the charge nurse had just one patient. Most of the time, he spent the shift outside, smoking weed or cigarettes. Otherwise, he was on the computer reading e-mails. He was useless. I saw the patient he had. He was a nice young man. Earlier, I helped him get to the phone to talk to his mom. He appeared in no distress at all at that time. Later that shift, I saw the nurse scrambling at his bedside. I didn't go in because I was stocked with patients where he had just the one.

Near the end of the shift, I walked by that patient's room to find the man blue and barely responsive with a high-flow oxygen mask on his forehead (a lot of good it did there). I called respiratory therapy to the ER, stat! I then moved the patient to the crash room and called the doctor in. He immediately intubated the patient. This young man lost his vital signs, no pulse, not breathing. We started CPR. As I was doing chest compressions, the charge nurse—his nurse—said goodnight. It was shift change, he was going home.

We continued the resuscitative efforts, but he died. Looking at the chart, the nurse started an IV and hung one liter of fluid. I guess it got away from him, so once it ran out he hung another, then another, then another. He was waiting for some blood products to arrive that he then infused. The patient received almost five liters of fluid in four hours. His lungs filled because his heart couldn't pump that much volume. Now, I don't have much of a poker face. I had no respect for this guy. The case was swept under the carpet.

Working triage again, a young girl was brought in by her parents. She wasn't alert and was suffering from severe dehydration. She reminded me of the girl who died years ago on Christmas Eve. I brought her back immediately, gathered IV supplies, and told another charge nurse about the patient. That nurse said, "Oh, she can go to the clinic. They can take care of her there." What? This patient was sick! I went into the patient's room to find that they were gone. I couldn't believe it!

Back in triage, I could hear some noise. I saw a pediatrician with the girl in his arms. He and the parents were running down the hall back into the ER. I met them with the IV supplies. I got the line, gave fluids, checked her blood sugar, and found it was 40 mg/dl. We gave some D25 IV, and the little girl did great. The charge nurse was promoted to nursing supervisor.

One of the nurses, Mona, was planning a "girls' night." I guess they were all going to get together for a good time. The invitation requested a song list for some karaoke. Well, I thought I'd list some songs as a joke. I listed "Soul Man," "I'm a Man," "Ramblin' Gamblin' Man." You get the picture. Every song that had "man" in the title. Most of us had a good laugh. Well, when Mona came in the next day, she was pissed! She hunted me down, got right up into my face, and warned me that if I added one more song, she would make my life hell. She meant it. It's fair to say our relationship never recovered. She was another one of those mean, lazy nurses with an attitude.

I walked into a room one day. The patient's wife asked me if I would brush her husband's teeth. She already asked Mona, who informed her that she was an ER nurse and didn't brush teeth. I told the lady I was happy to do so. I was an ER nurse, too, and I could brush teeth. That lady brought in four dozen doughnuts the very next day. In that same room, another patient asked me if I could elevate the head of his bed. He told me that Mona said the bed did not go up. I elevated the head of the bed for the patient, and he was more comfortable.

Later, I walked in the room where Mona was working. She was perplexed, as was the doctor beside her. They had a patient hooked up on a cardiac monitor but could not get a wave to appear. I looked at the patient, the lead wires, then the monitor. The monitor was set on a paddle lead and not the normal lead 2. I switched the channel on the monitor and the cardiac waveform appeared. Simple! The doctor said it was nice working with a real ER nurse. How well would that go over with Mona? Not very.

The next day, when I was working in triage, the husband of one of the nurses came in and sat beside me. He said, "Why don't you quit? You know none of us like you here." I responded that I wasn't there for a popularity contest. At just that moment, a patient arrested in the crash room. I walked in as they performed CPR. Mona was attempting to defibrillate the patient without success. The patient remained in V-fib. Mona handed me the paddles, asking if I wanted to try. I said sure.

I charged the paddles, yelled clear, pressed the paddles firmly on the patient's chest, and shocked her. The patient converted to a normal rhythm and regained a pulse. It was great, but Mona was miffed. She said, "Well, you just pressed harder." Now, the book says 25 pounds of pressure is to be applied to each paddle during defibrillation. If she knew that, perhaps she would have been successful. I was wondering how many patients died while under her nursing care, or lack thereof.

As time went on, things became even more difficult for me. It was a Friday night, and a seven-year-old boy came in short of breath and running a fever. An x-ray revealed he had whited out his entire left lung as a result of infection. The admitting doctor was paged. I picked up the phone and asked the pediatrician to come down. He wanted to know what was going on. I told him all the relevant information about the patient, and he said, "I don't believe it," then hung up the phone. I never saw him come down. The patient was sick, so I got him IV antibiotics and fluids.

At the same time, an obese black female was placed in the other bed. Both beds in the crash room were full now. She was severely short of breath as a result of acute congestive heart failure. She was cold, soaking wet, and breathing fast. I was almost certain she was going to die, so I moved as fast as I could. She needed everything we could throw at her to get all the fluid off her lungs and heart: morphine, nitroglycerine, and Lasix. All these meds would dilate her blood vessels and create room for the fluid to pool away from her heart and lungs, and also get her to pee a lot of it off.

As I grabbed more supplies in the med room, an ER technician entered. He came up behind me, slipped three fingers up into my anus, and said, "You know none of us like you, why don't you quit?" I told him I was too busy, but he kept on. I then encouraged him to gather his friends, so we could discuss it after work. My shift ended at 23:45. I was thinking about how my martial arts instructor would have us fight three-on-one when I was a kid. Now, I'm not generally overconfident, but I was very ready to find out.

The black lady did well. All the medicine did their job. She was warm, dry, and breathing normally, so I couldn't be happier. Her eyes were closed, and she was about to get an EKG. However, the respiratory therapist wanted to draw a blood gas beforehand, so the doctor could get information about how well the patient was oxygenating and ventilating. This required a needlestick in her radial artery. The therapist did not inform the lady she was about to get stuck and her eyes were closed. When the needle pierced her artery, she let out a very loud, "OWWW!!!"

I had something to say to the patient, and as far as I was concerned it was not for anyone else to hear. I got very close to her ear and whispered to her that the way she screamed she sounded just like James Brown!

Now, what happened next was one of the most defining moments in my nursing career. It was at that point that I realized nursing at its best is an art. You see, just a few moments before, the patient was cold, short of breath, and on the verge of death. Our little secret now had her laughing so hard, she almost flew off the gurney. What I whispered had her out of control. No one knew what was going on, and the EKG was full of artifact. She lost it. I'd never been so proud. I loved nursing! The shift was over. I walked outside only to find that the ER technician and his friends were nowhere to be found. I was a bit disappointed, as I was hoping for resolution.

CHAPTER 20

UNBELIEVABLE

I arranged for time with my manager. When I saw her, I said to her, "You know, I'm dealing with a lot here."

She replied, "Not many people like you here. If you choose to stay, you're going to have to find a way to deal with it." I was good with that.

I came in the next day through the ambulance entrance. There, I was greeted by the ER technician. He came up and bumped into my shoulder. I said, "Hey, why don't we go see the manager?"

We walked into the office and all I had to say was, "I'm going to ask you to stop touching and pushing me, okay? In fact, if you would just leave me alone, feel free to help the other nurses. I would just like to work in peace." I asked if he had any questions or if I could clear anything up. That was about it. I then walked out of the office and began my shift.

The next day, I was summoned back into administration to read a report stating I was yelling at the top of my lungs, about to assault the technician in front of my manager. The report stated the manager was ordering me to stand down and I was insubordinate! I was suspended for three days without pay and was required to attend an anger management course as a condition of future employment. Now I was pissed. I could not believe that my manager wrote those lies about me. I was having none of it.

I did get in the anger class, and I was paid for the time. I learned some management techniques and observed that there were some pretty angry people out there.

At the beginning of one class, the instructor asked me if I was willing to share any experiences I had since the previous week. I was happy to do so. I told him about a golf shot I had in which the ball flew over the green. Instead of becoming angry, I assessed the situation, envisioned the next shot, and chipped in for a birdie! I told him that if I responded with anger, I would most likely have had made a bogey! I'm not sure he liked my story.

I called my union rep and told her that what had been written about me was a fabrication. She was blown away. Of course, she also knew all the characters in that ER, since she had had many dealings with them in the past. I told her I would not lie down for it. I wanted my money back, I wanted out of the anger class, and I wanted my file clean! She fought, but it wasn't easy. I asked that she not give up on me, despite the fact that there was major pushback. She gave the case to the union big guy above her. From there, it went outside the hospital and into regional administration. There was no way I was backing down.

In triage again, my manager showed up. She said, "I didn't know you'd take it this far. Why didn't you talk to me, I would have given you your money back." I told her I wasn't comfortable talking to her without union representation and with that she left. I found her in the nursing lounge, curled on the couch in a fetal position, in tears. I told her I missed our friendship and agreed to drop everything if she returned my money, excused me from the anger class, and agreed to have the incident removed from my file. She confessed that she was coached into saying all those things about me by the HR representative.

I wondered about their character and integrity. It was painfully clear no cared about nurses.

The next day, my union representative had my check. I signed some papers and was good to go. As for the technician shoving me with his fingers in my ass—it was my word against his.

Sally was a wonderful lady, and I liked her a lot. She would show up in the ER regularly because she suffered from alcohol addiction. This time she was really sick, throwing up all kinds of bile. I was preparing to start an IV immediately when the brilliant Dr. Drew appeared. She was the doctor who believed she was smarter than everyone else; she was better educated after all.

Dr. Drew and I went way back, too. Suffice it to say, she was not often happy to see me. Years ago, I lost an earpiece to my stethoscope. She offered to give me one of her extra earpieces. She gave me her home address and invited me over to her place the next morning. I think she wanted to give me more than just an earpiece, but I never showed up. When I saw her years later, I was a bit taken aback. I was thinking, shit! I suspected our time together wasn't going to go well. It never did.

Anyway, Sally was vomiting, and Dr. Drew told me to give her a Compazine and morphine suppository to combat her nausea and pain. I didn't even know they made morphine suppositories. I thought the doctor was just being mean. I didn't know if this was directed at Sally, me, or possibly both. After a bit, I found

Sally on the floor, writhing in pain and vomiting bile everywhere. I called Dr. Drew in to look. She then told me to start the IV and give the meds immediately. That was a Friday night.

I came back to work Monday. The charge nurse asked me if I'd heard about Sally. I said no. He told me Sally had died and relayed that both he and Dr. Drew high-fived each other at the news. Evidently, they said, "We won't be seeing that fucking bitch here anymore!" I looked around the ER and felt nauseous. I don't pretend to be perfect. I'm most certainly not, but I was convinced that this was no place for me. There was something very wrong in this ER, and I didn't want to be around these people.

I was often back working in triage because the staff didn't want me in the ER with them; believe me, I was fine with that! A young lady came in complaining about some abdominal pain. I asked all the questions pertaining to her complaint, took her vitals, and sent her back into the ER. Moments later, the doctor approached me, grabbed my shoulders, and started to violently shake me. I stepped out of his grasp as he yelled, "Why didn't you tell me she had had an abortion?"

All I said was, "You got that information while speaking with her?" I was wondering who had the anger management issues. He was shaking me, which strained my neck. Somehow that was tolerated, and there was no consequence.

Sometimes patients just want to talk to the doctor. In their minds, the nurses are nobodies or maybe they are more comfortable behind a closed door with their doctor. I remember once at the old county hospital, I pulled young man out of the back of a car. He was wrapped in a blanket and he looked sick. I asked his mom if he had any medical problems. She said no! I grabbed the man, took him to the ER on a gurney, placed him on a cardiac monitor, took his vital signs, started an IV, and drew his blood. The doctor walked in and asked about his medical history. The first thing the mother said was, "Oh yes, he has AIDS!" How could a nurse ask the same question and get nothing? I remember that kid tossing and turning, he was so restless. He began bleeding from his eyes and mouth and died quickly.

Sometimes, it's fun to get a little payback! I knew a few things about Dr. Drew, including one of her weaknesses: sputum. Now, I'm a nurse and I can handle anything: blood, pus, stool, whatever. A patient arrived from a nursing home. She had a fever and her airway was compromised by a copious amount of sputum. I grabbed what they call a sputum trap and aggressively suctioned her airway. I was getting all kinds of thick, yellow sputum out of her, which we would call lung butter. It looked like custard! I collected the sample and was going to send it to the lab for culture. Before I sent it off, I figured a prudent nurse would have the physician assess the specimen. I mean, the doctor needed to know, right? Well as luck would have it, Dr. Drew was going to see the patient. However, she was busy sewing a laceration. As the good nurse that I was, I showed her the specimen by flashing it in front of her eyes while she was sewing. As she looked, there was a firing along the neural pathway from the optic nerve to the occipital lobe that then travelled to her frontal lobe, where some emotion was attached. It travelled further to her brainstem vomiting centers, coursed through her vagus nerve, fired into her abdomen, and resulted in reverse peristalsis. She was retching and about to vomit! I was tickled with the result. I was thinking your morphine suppository versus my sputum in your face. Touché.

CHAPTER 21

HOW MUCH MORE CAN YOU TAKE?

A new doctor was soon hired. I was optimistic but that didn't last long. Her name was Dr. Boston. It was clear that she carried a bit of arrogance. One thing I noticed over the years was that arrogance and competence tended to be inversely proportional.

I had a patient who was admitted for a large hematoma resulting from an angiography (a radiographic study of arterial blood flow), who bled from the catheter puncture of his femoral artery. He was a nice man in his 70s. I had him all worked up, he just needed a chest film.

I went down the hall to help a nurse get an IV started. Just as I was about to make the puncture, Dr. Hope asked me to get my patient to x-ray immediately. I could see by the look on her face that immediately meant immediately. The IV had to wait.

When I entered my patient's room, I met his daughter. She demanded to speak to my manager and threatened to sue me as well as the hospital for delaying her father's chest film. I told her that I was unaware of my manager's location at the time and directed her to the front desk to have her paged. The daughter was having none of it. She wanted me to find the manager. I again referred her to the front desk, telling her I could not do so. Just as I turned away to wheel her father to x-ray, I heard a threatening and deep voice. The son-in-law of the patient said, "Hey, don't start that!" It sounded like he was about to start a fight.

I turned back around, took off my glasses and stethoscope, and asked, "Or what?" Staring, he had nothing to say.

I then took the man to x-ray and went back to start the IV for my friend. In no time at all, I saw the x-ray technician running full stride back to the ER with the patient. Dr. Boston was there. A nurse was about to inject some medication into his IV, so I asked what he was injecting. He said Benadryl. I asked why, and he said, "I don't know." He then pushed it into the IV. Dr. Boston was screaming that the patient was having an anaphylactic reaction. I wanted more information. Another nurse had a syringe with epinephrine. I covered the IV port with my hand and wouldn't let him give it. I told the nurse the injection of epinephrine would kill the patient. I then looked at the x-ray tech and asked if she gave the patient any contrast dye. She said no! I turned to the patient, put him on the cardiac monitor, gave him some oxygen, and asked him to take some deep breaths. He was fine, he was just a bit anxious. Dr. Boston would have killed him.

As I rolled the man upstairs, he thanked me for everything. He said he knew how hard the service industry could be. He saw his daughter threaten to sue me, his son-in-law nearly pick a fight, and watched as I jumped in front of the staff who would have killed him. I told him, "Don't worry about me, just get well and get out of here!"

As I walked past the crash room, I could see Dr. Boston at the bedside of a patient. I'm not sure why I walked in there. The patient looked alert. He didn't appear to be in any distress, but I noticed that his skin was pretty mottled. The condition of his skin is often representative of poor blood delivery and oxygen uptake—not a good sign. I asked Dr. Boston if she was going to intubate the patient. In her condescending fashion, she asked, "Why would I do that?"

No sooner, the patient had a V-fib arrest. We started CPR and I said, "Well, I guess you'll intubate him now!"

Later the same day, a man came in after ingesting an unknown quantity of Vicodin, Valium, and vodka. He wanted to die. The man lost his wife to breast cancer. Overcome with the loss, pain, and grief, he was not in a place where he could effectively cope.

I explained to the patient and his son that the doctor (Dr. Boston) had ordered gastric lavage, which meant putting a tube down into his stomach to pump out what he had taken. I restrained him, not for punishment, but to keep him from pulling the tube.

Now, the patient fought like hell and was vomiting all over. I was struggling to place the tube and keep his airway clear with suction. I decided the procedure was not safe and informed Dr. Boston. As an alternative, I suggested paralytics and intubation to get it done. She scowled at me and said, "Get another nurse!" I gave report to another nurse and walked to the minor care clinic. I twisted my back during the struggle and thought I'd better get it documented.

When I returned to the department, I noticed my patient was gone! His daughter approached me, demanding my name and the nursing supervisor. Next thing I know, my manager was called. She had me in the office and asked me what was going on. I told her about attempting the lavage, giving report to the other nurse, going to the clinic, then returning to find the room empty. She told me that my story differed from the daughter's. The daughter said that I watched and laughed as her father eloped, exclaiming that this is how we like to take care of our patients here!

I was told that there would be a meeting with administration the following day and that I'd better have my union representative with me. I told the manager, I wasn't even in the department. She didn't care; she would not listen to me. Well, I did one better. I went to the security office and secured a copy of the surveillance tape. The hallway film showed no evidence of my presence at the time the patient ran off. I was cleared. I loved being an ER nurse. I went to school and got the job I dreamed of. Now, I had a family to support, but this was becoming unbearable.

It was now shift change, but before leaving another overdose patient arrived. The staff made no effort to go into the room and assess the patient as he was. Instead of leaving the department, I placed the patient on a cardiac monitor, started an IV, and drew labs. Still no one came by, so I placed the gastric tube, evacuated his stomach, and administered charcoal. I placed a Foley catheter and sent his urine off to the lab for a toxicology report. No one ever came in the room, not one doctor came to assess this guy. I charted my interventions, finally gave report to a nurse, and left. I was prepared to be called in the office and fired. I really didn't care. I figured if I ended up in front of a judge and jury, I'd have my day in court. This place was horrible.

I went back into work the next day. I had seven patients, one of whom was pulled out of the ambulance entrance and I was buried with orders. I sat to do some charting when an orthopedic technician asked me to come down and help move a patient. I asked him to please get the ER tech or charge nurse because I was too behind.

Moments later, the manager came up to me. I was accused of refusing to help while I was on the phone making personal calls.

She said I was endangering patients by delaying care. I challenged her to provide dates and times when care was delayed. I then made her a deal. I said I would quit if I received no negative reference from this place. She agreed. I handed over my badge and just like that, I quit! I wasn't nervous about it. I still had the job at the mini-county hospital, and I landed a pretty good side job working for an ambulance company. I'd be fine.

The mini-county hospital staffed the ER with family medicine doctors at times. It was difficult for me to wrap my head around that. I figured emergency rooms should have board-certified emergency room doctors, but what do I know?

I was walking by a trauma room to find a woman who was in an accident that resulted in a car fire. I peaked in and could see her face was burnt and blistered. She had a hoarse cough, and there was black around her mouth. The family medicine doctor was leaving the room, and I asked him if he was going to intubate the patient. He replied by asking, "Why would I do that?"

And just like so many years ago, I replied "If I were you, I'd intubate her while you still have the chance!" He went back in there and tubed the patient.

He chased me down after and thanked me, noting her airway was close to be swollen shut. He asked how I knew. I told him that I read a book. I was getting a bit tired of emergency rooms and began to think perhaps I would fare better on my own. Accordingly, I made myself more available for the ambulance work. I would have more autonomy, more responsibility, and I would be largely out of the hospital.

CHAPTER 22

TAKE TO THE HIGHWAY, TAKE TO THE AIR

The ambulance proved to be just the ticket. I liked being on my own. I worked with a couple EMTs who were kids with a teaspoon of education and a license to drive the ambulance. Most of them were on their way to becoming firefighters or paramedics.

It was interesting to work with them. Some of the EMTs were sharp. They had their eyes and ears open, and they needed no direction. Others displayed a bit of arrogance, thinking they saw and knew it all. I had to watch those guys. Still others had a disdain for nurses. I would find some of them harbored resentment, though for what I had no clue. My salary was often a topic with them. I replied, "Go to school!" We started our days around 5 AM. Most of the early morning calls were into the city. We transferred patients who needed large medical center specialty services, often cardiac cases.

We had to be ready for anything. Some patients were awake, alert, and totally stable. Others were on ventilators and medications requiring blood pressure support. We ran one call and waited for the next. Some days were incredibly busy, and others allowed us to hang by the oceanside sipping on lattes and enjoying bagels with cream cheese. It was a good job.

At times, nurses would strike, which meant we had to move all their ICU patients out to other nearby medical centers. Those days could last up to 24 hours. Call after call, I got tired.

One day, we were moving patients. As we prepared to leave the hospital parking lot, the EMT I was with saw his girlfriend in another ambulance. He had to say hello. He jumped in her rig. The doors closed, and time passed. The van was rocking, and I didn't go knocking. They needed their time. I found a local coffee shop and 30 minutes later, I returned. We then proceeded to our next call.

One particular summer day, we were driving along the coast into a small beach town. I noticed a cute young lady walking her dog. She was wearing shorts, had long legs, and was licking an ice-cream cone. It was a sight to behold. An EMT named Mike was driving the rig as I pointed her out to him. Mike was completely mesmerized, but what he failed to notice was that the Oldsmobile in front of us had stopped and was backing into a parking place! I screamed, "STOP!" The ambulance was a big box rig and it was slamming back and forth, back and forth trying to stop. We missed the car's rear end by inches. The girl walked past us with the biggest grin on her face! She knew!

I began to realize how pathetic nursing was everywhere. We arrived at the sending hospital to pick up a patient; they couldn't wait to get the patient out of there. When we arrived at the receiving hospital, we were invisible. No one wanted to admit him. I remember being a kid and looking at hospitals thinking the smartest people in the world worked there! The fall off that pedestal would meet trauma center criteria! It had become unfathomable, the degree of apathy and incompetence I had begun to recognize.

Despite it all, I still liked the job. They were happy with me at the ambulance company because I worked and would come in anytime. When I wasn't working, I loved playing golf. The annual membership was due at my local course, and I really didn't want to spend the money. I walked in to work and said to Lena, my boss, "I want a $500 bonus. I deserve it and I want it." She told me to hold on and returned with a check for $500. I had free golf for a year! Sometimes you just have to ask!

I saw a fax come through the office from an air medical company looking for nurses. I thought I would apply and give it a shot. I knew a few nurses who flew, and they were cool. I noticed that some of the flight nurses had a bit of an attitude, which I didn't completely understand. I figured if there was someone with a rocket launcher trying to blow you out of the sky, then you had balls! If not, you were just another transport nurse who got around in a faster ambulance with no stop signs. The only real difference was that there was less chance of surviving a crash when you fall out of the sky.

I went in for the interview, which was something! They threw everything at me: pediatric stuff, airway management, trauma! I was fielding every question and noticed I'd begun to sweat. It reminded me of the time I was in my high school principal's office for jumping through the bus window trying to get a free ride! The last question was, "What would you give if your patient became tachycardic while on a nitroprusside drip?" I looked at him and said Inderal. I didn't blink! I got the job and I was psyched! They told me nobody scored as high as I did on their entrance exam. I remember thinking that old county hospital ER job really paid off!

The first day of training was with my supervisor on the fixed wing. While we made introductions, I could see he was tired. Apparently, he had been up flying all night. I said, "Not too much sleep, huh?"

He replied, "Fuck you!" Those words never sat well with me. Instead, I put my head down, took some breaths, and kept telling myself, "You want this job!" It was a lesson learned from the movie *Back to the Future*. When someone called Marty McFly a chicken and he responded with anger, nothing ever went well for him. I learned from McFly!

We began the training. I learned a lot about flight nursing and safety procedures. The equipment included all the stuff I had been working with on the ambulance, so I breezed through the ventilators, IV pumps, and cardiac monitors. I was in and I was ready to go! I was about to have the time of my life! The doctor who owned and ran the operation was incredible! He was smart, energetic, filled with passion, and he had a mission. I loved the guy, he was fair, he was tough, and he was gruff! He took no shit, it was his boat! He reminded me of my grandfather.

Before long, I was flying all the time, both on the fixed wing and the rotor wing (helicopter). I preferred the fixed wing. The flights were longer, and the seats were like La-Z-Boys. The rotor wing was small, fast, and loud. It vibrated all the time. We used it to respond to 911 emergencies also.

There is a hierarchy of egos in medicine and nursing. At the top are the neurosurgeons, cardiovascular surgeons, and the anesthesiologists. Beneath them are the general surgeons, cardiologists, and intensivists. The ER doctor is at the bottom, and I'm not too sure where family medicine or pediatricians fit. Now, nursing plays at the same game. First of all, everyone dumps on nursing, everyone! Within nursing, the cardiac ICU nurses are at the top, then it's the neurosurgical ICU nurses, followed by the surgical and medical ICU nurses. Again, the ER nurses hover at the bottom, while medical surgical nurses and clinic nurses don't even count. OR nurses aren't really nursing, they just count stuff and look at the patient's chart. The paramedics in the field dump on the EMTs. Still, nursing takes the biggest hit from everyone—administration, doctors, nurses, medics, everyone! But flight nurses are true superheroes.

My supervisor, Mr. "FU," is an ICU nurse. I've only ever considered myself an ER nurse, although I have worked in a number of critical care departments over the years. Anyhow, we had discussions. While he knew more ICU stuff, I noted that in the ER I saw the patient first, put in the lines and tubes, and assisted in the life-saving procedures. Only once they were stable did they go to the ICU nurse. All they did was watch the monitor and titrate the IV drips I started. I left it at that. Now honestly, I didn't care but he was always bringing the shit up. So, whenever we got a baby to transfer, I'd ask him if he wanted to start the IV. Those sorts of things were left to me, obviously!

One day, we were sent out for an advanced trauma class. He took the class before, but it was my first time. The ICU nurse was going on and on about how hard it was going to be. I always studied hard and put in all the effort I could. I told him I wasn't worried since I'd spent 10 years in a trauma center! I had a ball. I was putting in chest tubes, surgical Cricothyrotomies, venous cutdowns, subclavian lines. I was doing every possible procedure that I could.

When the test was administered, I was the first to complete it. I breezed through the clinical, and during my exit interview I was told I scored 100 percent. They asked me to come on board as a trauma nurse instructor! While the offer was nice, I was away from home quite a bit already. I declined. As I came out of the room, my supervisor, the ICU nurse, asked me how I did. I told him, "You don't want to know."

As we returned to our base, I saw Dr. Mack. He asked me about my time in Texas at the course. I told him I had a good time. He then asked what grade I got. I looked him straight in the eye and said, "I got the grade I wanted."

He grinned and said, "I think you got the grade everyone wanted." We both had the best laugh!

The doctor always kept our skills sharp. We were always training and being tested. He particularly enjoyed picking on me! Though there were 75 employees, he was always asking me the questions. One day he asked us, "Why do we give oxygen?"

Around the room, people were giving the obvious answers, "The patient is hypoxic," "The patient's O2 saturation is low," etc. None of them were correct.

The doctor repeated, "Why do we give oxygen?"

Finally, I raised my hand and said, "Because oxygen is the final electron acceptor at the end of the electron transport chain that occurs on the folds of the mitochondria called the cristae."

He responded, "Now that's the answer I'm looking for!" People were shaking their heads. All I did was recall a test question from a microbiology class 15 year earlier!

I loved flight nursing because it pushed my knowledge base and skills to the maximum. It was fun, challenging work, just like it was back at the old county hospital!

Back on the ground, however, the luster was being lost. The kids driving the ambulance flew over speed bumps and sent me up into the air while I was working in the back. It was fun for them. When I was flying, I didn't have to deal with children. It was professional. The doctor had no room or tolerance for jerks. I preferred to fly, and it was nonstop travel!

CHAPTER 23

FIRING ON ALL CYLINDERS

Dr. Mack ran the flight program like the military. We were training all the time. He had a love for children, so we were always reviewing pediatric emergencies, trauma, and more about airway management.

I had a call to a small rural hospital. The patient was a seven-week-old infant who had only been out of the ICU for a week and needed to get back to the medical center in the city. My partner and I arrived to find a four-kilogram baby in respiratory distress. He was sick. His respiratory rate was 70 and so was his O2 saturation. We had orders to sedate, intubate, and transfer.

Now, the staff tried to gain IV access numerous times, and what I gathered was that the doctor attempted an intraosseous (bone) needle insertion six times! That's when you place a needle right into the patient's tibia bone. This baby looked like swiss cheese! My partner and I discussed our plan. I drew up the Versed, and we got our airway stuff together. I told my partner he had one chance at the tube, then I would take over. I tied the kid's arm off with a tourniquet, said a prayer, and stuck him with a 24 g

IV. I got a flash of blood and threaded the catheter into the vein. I was in! I then pushed the Versed as my partner dropped in the tube. We had the airway. I dialed in our ventilator and we were good to go!

The hospital staff applauded us. They were so happy that they loaded us up with chips, soda, and juice. All the while, I was telling them we couldn't carry it. They were so elated they escorted us out to the plane! We got the baby to the city. It was a good moment.

When we first arrived on the scene, I knew it was going to be serious and challenging work. I was hoping that whatever we did we would not kill the patient. As I reflect on it now, I don't know how I did it. The truth is that the years I spent at the old county pediatrics ER prepared me for that very moment. I attribute much of it to the incredible Dr. Mary. I was so fortunate to work beside her. She pushed me then to become a better nurse. Truth be told, she still inspires me today.

A good partner is also key. I worked with Brian and every call was a blast. We had fun, pushed each other, and had each other's back. I also worked with Jane, which was a different experience. She was a know-it-all. She had previous experience working trauma and spent time in the ER of the general hospital. She tended to go on about everything she had done. In short, she was full of herself.

I found her to be lazy and basically careless. One particular incident that comes to mind involved a two-year-old patient who had had a seizure followed by respiratory arrest. I was calling out for some drugs based on the patient's weight. Jane was handing me incorrect doses and instructing me to give them anyway! I couldn't believe it. She was more of a hindrance than anything else.

Another medic I worked with wasn't much better. I think he was more into the title of flight medic. He clearly wasn't too concerned with patient care. Most of his stories during our flights revolved around his sexual adventures. Our flight times would be filled of anecdotes about the girls he was with and what they would do. I was much past 16 years of age, so the stories didn't hold much interest to me. I had a daughter and hoped she'd never meet a yo-yo like him. I grew so tired of him, I basically told him to just shut up.

Our tension was noticeable and eventually we were directed to work out our differences by the flight program director. I swallowed my pride and we worked it out to an extent. All the while, I was wondering if the flight director had any idea about what this medic was saying about her!

My other partner was very experienced and loved flight nursing. She was invested in the procedures and very emotional. I worked hard with her on every call.

One Saturday, we had a full day. It began with a call to the beach. Five people were dead. Their boat capsized and there was nothing we could do. We received another call. A bicyclist crashed, and her hip was broken. We packed her up and flew her to the trauma center. We got a call about another bicycle crash. The rider had no helmet and was unresponsive. We intubated him and travelled back to the trauma center!

Now we were off to a hospital. A man crashed his motorcycle, and he was in their ICU on a ventilator. IV lines were everywhere. The patient was 250 pounds, and all messed up. He had pulmonary contusions (bruising and blood clots in his lungs). I switched him over to our ventilator, changed the IV tubing to fit our IV pumps, and zeroed his arterial and CVP lines (internal lines that measured his blood pressure and blood volume status). We loaded him up in the helicopter and away we went.

I was suctioning blood clots out of his endotracheal tube constantly. It was already mid-afternoon, and we had yet to eat! After the call, we were able to get some food and things quieted down for a bit. It eventually got dark and we received a call that took us out deep into the woods. We found a man who was drunk. He fell out of his wheelchair and into his campfire. He couldn't get out, he was stuck and began to BBQ himself. When we arrived, I was met by an old friend, who was the paramedic on scene. I started the IV line, pushed some morphine to relieve the patient's pain, loaded the patient up to then off the trauma center. I wanted to take him directly to the burn center, but we had to go to the closest facility.

Once we arrived at the trauma center, an ER nurse started screaming, "We use Lactated Ringer's on our burn patients!" I was blown away by her antics. I hung normal saline because that's what we carried in our limited helicopter supply room, which was the side pocket in the door.

We were called back to the trauma center in 45 minutes to transfer the patient to the burn center (where I wanted to go in the first place). As I entered the room, I found the patient naked on the gurney. The IV was dry, and he was shivering! I guess that's how they treat their burn patients! The moment we dropped him off, we received another call about a drunk driver. The passenger was ejected from the vehicle. We got to a remote area that we could access and waited there as an ambulance brought the patient to us. They arrived 45 minutes later, they were performing CPR. The car flipped, crushing the victim's head! She was dead. She had been dead a long time, but my procedure-hungry partner had to intubate. I was begging her to call it and leave, but she couldn't help herself. We opened everything and did all we could, but the victim remained dead. I had to restock everything.

It was 3 AM I was spent and needed some sleep. We received another call about a 45-year-old man who flipped his car off the freeway. As we arrived, we saw an ambulance and a fire engine on the scene. The victim was surrounded. He was spewing blood like a volcano. The first responders were trying to intubate but couldn't visualize his airway. I decided to do a crich!

I grabbed a scalpel, made an incision over his trachea, then cut his cricothyroid membrane, making a hole where the tube could fit. The victim's pulse became weaker and began to slow. I started an IV, pushing fluids and epinephrine. The victim arrested. We began CPR, working frantically to save his life. He died in a cold, dark field at 5 AM on a Sunday morning.

I was spent, physically exhausted, and emotionally drained. The day had been nothing but blood and death from beginning to end. We barely ate, and I barely slept. I was packing our stuff up when a police officer turned to me and said, "Nice job." I was about to freak out. He saw my face and backed up. Stepping back, he put his arms in the air and said, "No, I saw what you did. If I ever needed a nurse, I hope it's you who responds." All I could do was bow my head and hold back tears. It had been a long day. The next day, I was informed that the medic on scene was blaming me for killing the patient. I spoke with the doctor and gave him the blow-by-blow. He said we will wait to see what the coroner says.

I was thinking about the man who passed away. I was sleeping when he flew off the freeway and was ejected from his automobile. I was under the covers when his brain was slamming around the inside of his skull as his head hit the ground. A lot of energy was transferred during that deceleration and certainly none of that was my fault.

I thought about the amount of time he was out there exposed and hypothermic before 911 was called and the time it took firefighters and medics to respond and to eventually call me. I wondered why they didn't secure his airway and start IVs and transfer him to the nearby trauma center. How could this guy be blaming me?

The coroner's report was placed in my mailbox at work. It detailed a venous and arterial brain bleed, a torn artery in his lung, and aspiration of blood was revealed. The coroner did note that the tracheal tube was correctly positioned. I never heard another word about it.

My next shift, I almost died. We landed on a beach at night. A volunteer fireman met us there to drive us to the patient's house. I jumped in the truck and could smell alcohol on his breath. As I was in the cab going through our equipment bag, he began to drive. I could immediately sense something was wrong. The guy was driving towards the helicopter and almost crashed into the rotor blades! I screamed, "Stop!"

He said, "I'm pulling a U-turn, I can make it." I told him to look up, and as he did, he put the truck in reverse!

I really loved the job. I felt I would do it forever. Next to the position at the pediatrics ER, it was the best job I ever had.

I recalled one nurse I worked with in an ER who gave me grief about treating every patient like an emergency. On this job, I could do my thing with other skilled nurses. I had a nurse manager once tell me I cared too much, but now I was with a doctor who was passionate about our mission. Even if you made some sort of mistake, what mattered was that you were thinking about what was best for the patient. We all learned!

I worked there for a number of years and had a ball. Then the compensation structure changed. The first shift, I lost $135 in wages. By the second shift, I was down $150. I spoke to the program director about the lost income and the response was, "We are paying you $50K annually to be on call." They say liars' figure and figures lie. The truth is that I was down almost $300 in two days. As much as I hated to do it, I gave notice. I was getting a bit older, and I did not want to be working for less.

I figured I could get another job in a hospital and run calls on an ambulance, if needed. Then maybe, just maybe, I would walk away from nursing. I started looking for a job in the newspaper. As luck would have it, I got back on an ambulance and picked up a gig working for a plastic surgeon. My job was to sedate his patients while he was performing all sorts of revisions. It was easy money. I was working, and there was no BS! I was happy. I didn't miss hospital nursing. I was freelancing more or less, it worked for me.

CHAPTER 24

I WANT BACK IN

Working for the plastic surgeon was easy money. He called me in for a case. Occasionally, his hour-long case ended up lasting two or three hours. Once, I gave 1000 mcg of fentanyl and 15 mg of Versed during a procedure. This was way too much medication for me to be giving safely. It got me thinking that the plastic surgeon needed to spend more money for an anesthetist or an anesthesiologist. Someone who had more drugs and more airway skills would provide a safer environment for the patient. I did not like being in this indefensible position; it wasn't safe.

I was so relieved by my experience there it gave me a really good glimpse. My goal in the beginning of my nursing career was to become a nurse anesthetist, but my wife became pregnant with our third child. I stayed put in the ER since full-time school simply was not going to happen! What I had found was that putting people to sleep all day was incredibly boring. I thrived on the chaos the ER brought. Working in an ambulance was fine, but it could be a bit uncomfortable. It was common to get held over on calls and be kept long after the end of shifts; it was just the nature of the business.

My wife had a lump, and the mammogram was inconclusive. Her doctor wanted to take a biopsy to be sure. He said to me, "I don't know why I'm doing it, but if she was my wife I would." The results came back, and the news was not good. She had an appointment with a surgeon, but when we arrived we were told the surgeon called in sick. I was a bit upset that no one called us to reschedule. My wife gathered up the nerve for the appointment. Upon arriving, she was told to go home. I saw a picture on the wall of the clinic. It was of an old friend and surgeon from the old county days. I knocked on some office doors looking for him. Dr. Grand came out and greeted us. It was so good to see him. I told him why we were there and asked if he'd do me a favor. I told him I wanted him to take over my wife's care. He agreed immediately, stopped everything, and saw her right then and there.

The surgery was set. I knew the anesthesiologist and the scrub nurse. I loved them both. My old buddy was running the recovery room! Being on the other side, I got to see these people for who they were. I could not have handpicked a better team. They were angels. They donned scrubs every day and cared for the ill, the injured, the dying, and cared for their grieving, scared families. They were the best of human beings. I wanted so badly to be back among them.

It was a year before my wife was really back. It took two surgeries, chemotherapy, and weekly radiation treatments. She stayed strong through all of it, endured the pain, the hair loss, the nausea, and I'm glad to say she survived! She had a great medical and nursing team behind her.

I started putting my feelers out for another ER job. I really didn't want to return to the hospitals where I worked before, so I expanded my search. Getting online, I sent out an application.

Within 30 minutes, my phone rang. I was arranging an interview!

I met with the manager of the ER department. She seemed really nice. It was obvious that she had a military background, which I liked. Most of the time, those people are straight shooters. She invited another staff nurse into the interview process. It was safe to say they were interviewing me, but I was also interviewing them. The place was small with 10 beds in total. I thought that even if I was with a couple slug nurses, I couldn't be hurt too badly. After all, there were only 10 beds!

The interview process was going very well. I'd gained a lot of experience and my resume looked good. The staff nurse expressed one concern, though. She noticed I had been out of hospital nursing for six years and said that the nurses here tended to work on their own in the department. She was concerned about my ability to place nasogastric tubes and urinary catheters. I wanted to say, "Are you kidding me?" but I thought for a moment. I then turned to the manager and said, "Well I don't think human anatomy had changed in the last six years!" We all had a good laugh. I got the job! I was back working in an ER. I was good to go!

The place got pretty busy, which helped me to hit my stride. I was having a good time being back in the saddle. The staff seemed pretty cool and tight-knit. They'd known each other for years. The doctors were pretty close, too. They all completed their residencies together and staffed the ER as a group for the previous 20 years or so.

The manager really liked me, which was nice. She pulled me into her office one day and said that she was happy with my charting. She went on to note, "I'm really surprised. I always hear something negative about staff, but I'm hearing nothing negative about you!" I thought that was nice. I also wondered how long that would last!

My mom called and told me she had some difficult news. She said she had lung cancer, which had spread into her brain. Now, my mom told me she was going to quit smoking ever since I was a kid. She never did until she got the diagnosis.

I talked to my manager and asked if I could give up my shifts. I told her about my mom and she cleared my schedule. She said my family was more important and the hospital would still be standing.

When I got to my mom, I could see how sick she'd become. I decided that there was no way I could leave her and go back home. My five-day trip lasted a month. She looked at me and said, "I brought this on myself." I had nothing to say. She was right, and now she was dying. I was losing my mother because of cigarettes.

She was being discharged from the hospital as I waited in the car in front of the building. The snow was mixed with freezing rain. As I was waiting for my sister to bring our mom down, a security guard tapped my window. He was ordering me to move along. I told him I was waiting for my mom. He replied the elevators take forever and again told me to move. I was trying to appeal to his good nature and told him I was taking my mother home to die, but he was adamant I move. When I refused, he threatened to bring in his manager. They both began to team up on me. I got out of the car yelling at them that there was no way I was moving this car. About that time, my sister appears with our mom, she's completely hunched over in a wheelchair. I could see the embarrassment and the shame on the security officers faces. They helped my mom into the car carefully, and I thanked them for their help.

Back in her home, I cared for her the best I could. I tried to keep her comfortable and pain-free. One day, she looked at me and said, "I don't know what I would ever have done without you."

I replied, "Well mom, I don't know what I would ever have done without you." We looked at each other and I asked, "We square?"

"We're square," she said.

Wrapped in the arms of morphine, she fell asleep. On that Monday morning, she never woke. I was grateful that I could care for her as a loving son who was equipped as a nurse. I thought that this was one of my greatest nursing moments. I got back home and returned to the ER. I found it a bit of a challenge. I had no real time to grieve my loss because I was too busy helping others.

There were times I drove home, passing the field where I landed in a helicopter years before. I thought of the man who died in that field and what the police officer said to me. I missed talking to my mom. I dried my tears before I got home.

CHAPTER 25

SOME SUNDAY MORNINGS

I grew up going to church on Sundays, so I always felt Sunday mornings were sacred. Sunday mornings in the ER are anything but.

I walked into work and found a patient tied to the gurney. IVs were running, and the urinary catheter was in place. He was out of it. I got report and it turns out he was partying and ended up in the ER. Once there, he became extremely violent. He was so aggressive, the staff had to medicate him and put him out. When I came on, he had been there for over eight hours. I figured he had enough rest, and it was time for him to be discharged.

I shook him, and he woke easily. I explained I would be disconnecting everything, so he could go home. I asked who I could call to get him. I then took out the urinary catheter, untied his restraints, and told him I'd be back in a moment.

I could hear Sandy, my co-worker, screaming. I walked back in the room. The patient had ripped out his IV and was bleeding everywhere. He was standing up on the gurney looking crazed.

Sandy was scared. I asked what was going on, and the patient jumped at me. I jumped up in the air to meet him, wrapped my arm around his neck, and locked the hold with my other arm. I had secured him in what the MMA fighters would call a guillotine! Sandy screamed, "You're going to break his neck!" I told her to call a code gray! When a code gray is called, all the guys in the hospital come out of the woodwork. Now, this was good for me because I wasn't too sure how long it would be before I would run out of gas. Soon, this guy's arms could be around my neck!

I was a bit frustrated. We succeeded in getting the guy tied back down, but he was still raging. I was thinking of my friends who were already in church and here I was sweating. I called the police. This guy needed to go. The police arrived to take him, and now they were in a fight. The guy was saying things to those officers that one should never say. In the struggle, his gown was torn to shreds. I offered paper scrubs since he was now completely exposed. The guy told me to go fuck myself and was then cuffed. He was escorted to the police cruiser and taken to the city jail completely naked. Five minutes later, his brother showed up to take him home. He knew he was too late. I could see the sadness on his face.

Somehow, I was reminded of a time I had done a PM shift at the pit hospital I had quit years before. They were short for their next AM shift, which was a Sunday. They begged me to come in, which meant doubling back. In other words, I would get off at midnight, sleep, and be back to work by seven in the morning. I have always struggled to say no, so I agreed. Walking in the next morning, eyes still burning, I was met by nurse Mona. I'm sure she was thrilled to see me. Her first words were, "Did you get any sleep?" She was just trying to needle me. She was in charge that morning, which meant that her girlfriend would be sent to triage, where there would not be any patients for hours. There were two patients in the ER. One was going home (she took this patient) and one was being admitted (mine, of course). Otherwise it was quiet, so I was going to do what I needed to do to get through the day. I was having some coffee, still trying to wake up, and Mona could not stay off my back. She said, "I want you to go through the crash room checklist." I sipped my coffee and she asked, "Well, are you?"

I replied, "No, I'm going to just sit here and read my e-mails all day."

I was in the crash room doing the checklist when Mona told me the manager was on the phone! I took the call and the manager asked me what was wrong. Now I looked at Mona asking, "You called her?' I was blown away, she called the boss at 7:05 on a Sunday morning. I told my boss everything was fine, and I'd give a good day's work. We hung up. I then turned to Mona and told her that I wanted to give her my mother's phone number, so she could call her, too! You should have seen her face! She wasn't really a nurse, she was more of a monster.

Another Sunday, I was working with Tracy. Tracy was awesome. She was smart, experienced, and fun. I always looked forward to working with her. Every day was good. The paramedic radio went off and we were getting a lady who had been found down. The patient arrived out of sorts, so Tracy and I worked together. After some time, she came around. She was awake and appeared to be in no distress. Her family was beside her, and I was happy to see that. We served her breakfast, and all was well. Tracy saw the patient out.

The ER was getting busy and all the beds were full. Tracy approached me and said the patient she sent out had to come back. I told her I would get a bed. Moments later, Tracy told me that the patient was unresponsive. I looked at her and could see her concern. The patient was in the passenger seat of the car, by the ambulance entrance. We headed out there with a gurney. I opened the door and the patient made no response. I checked her carotid artery, and she was pulseless. I turned to Tracy saying, "Unresponsive? I think she's dead!" Somehow, I lifted this woman out of the car. We got her on the gurney and started CPR! Trying to get back into the ER, we realized that the code to the ambulance bay door had been changed. We didn't have it, so we crashed through the door! We had gotten the patient back in the ER on a monitor. She was in V-fib, so the doctor placed an IO (intraosseous) needle in her leg to give epinephrine. It wouldn't push. We placed another IO and pushed the epinephrine, but it was spouting out the first hole! I was fishing for a vein and got one. We gave more medication, continued CPR, and defibrillated numerous times.

She died. I couldn't believe it. I looked up to see the doctor in tears. Sad.

CHAPTER 26

CONTROL FREAKS

Now, it can easily be said that most nurses are control freaks, but the funny thing about control is you really have none. The way I look at it is that we're all on a blue marble spinning around a star suspended in infinity. What's more, we never know what's going to happen when we're working in an ER! Every nurse needs to learn to adapt rapidly to changing conditions, prioritize, and hopefully you are prepared!

Our ER manager had left, and we were working without one for quite some time. Lilly was often in charge of the ER, and she was a textbook control freak. It was almost laughable. I quickly noticed that anytime there was an emergency, she would be found at the foot of the bed! Managing emergencies almost always required being at the head of the bed, where she would never be found, perhaps because it was out of her control.

One day, she was in triage and getting backed up, so I took a chart off the wall, brought a patient back, and began the workup. Lilly came running back, chased me down, and asked what I had done. She began screaming at me, saying, "I need to know what's going on back here!"

I thought it was a bit odd because I was only trying to help, and there were only 10 beds. It was not a difficult ER to manage. I just shut my mouth and said, "Okay."

Not 10 minutes later, Lilly came up to me asking if I could grab another patient to triage since she was getting behind!

Diane came in to work with us. She was a traveler nurse and was obviously a bit older than the crew. She lived and breathed ER nursing. I liked her quite a bit.

Once, Diane made the fatal error of writing on our board. What's worse, she had written the patient's chief complaint in red marker! Lilly saw what Diane had done and she tore into her like I had never seen. I watched a young lady verbally assault her elder, a mature professional woman who could have easily been her mother. It was disgusting.

It was April Fools' Day, and I could see Diane walking up the driveway. I asked the clerk to nod when Diane was about to enter the ER. I had drawn the drapes around the gurney in our crash room. I got the signal and began doing CPR on a pillow. I screamed to the clerk "Call a code blue!" Diane ran into the room, tore the curtains open, and saw me resuscitating a pillow laughing my ass off! She slammed me against the wall and began to slap the shit out of me. I couldn't stop laughing. It was the best April Fools' joke ever!

I enjoyed working in that ER and wanted to stay. Even so, wars were breaking out over the schedule, and nurses have a real thing about their work schedules! Lilly had an ongoing battle with the scheduling coordinator. The sad thing was that before the conflict began, the assistant manager would do all scheduling. Things ran smoothly. Once Lilly got control of the scheduling, she planned a meeting at her house to build a workable schedule for everyone. I was disinclined to go. Her house was the last place I wanted to be on a day off. As a consequence, all the nurses got their dream schedule. I noticed that my days changed, and I would be working every other day. I saw it and said it wouldn't work for me.

I was in a situation where I would never enjoy any time off because I was either working until 7 PM or back to work at 7 AM. Lilly's response was, "Well, you didn't come to the meeting." Lilly had a schedule that worked with the schedule of her husband. The other nurses needed time for kids or other jobs. I drew the short straw, but I wasn't about to be under her thumb. I searched the job board and saw a day shift opening. They wanted a float nurse, one who could work in any department, give lunch breaks, and such. I applied and was moving out of the ER. Lilly got wind of it and demanded to know why I was leaving. I was not about to give her the answer. I was excited about the change. I was going to be able to set my own schedule, and I would be bouncing around everywhere. I thought it was going to be great!

CHAPTER 27

SOMETIMES, DEATH IS ALL AROUND

Sometimes things just don't make any sense. I received news that a nurse I worked with had killed herself. She'd lost her husband and her kids were out of control. She worked hard in the ER for years. I also heard that an ER doctor passed away. He was brilliant, one of the best I had known, but succumbed to AIDS. There was a nurse who arrived in the ER, having nearly done himself in with carbon monoxide by keeping his car running while parked in his garage with the door closed. Another friend and a phenomenal nurse overdosed on narcotics. Another ER doctor I knew died as he attempted to rescue a drowning victim.

As if this wasn't enough, I received more news that a helicopter crashed. The nurse that was killed was an angel and incredibly smart and gifted. She was among the best I had ever worked beside. Once, I tried recruiting her to work with us on our flight team. She looked at me and said she would never go up in one of those things, so I dropped it. When I found out that she was one of the nurses who died in the crash, I wondered who could have changed her mind?

I remembered one day when we were preparing to go out on a flight, the pilot had a bad look on her face. She looked like she'd lost her best friend. When I asked what was wrong, she told me she was looking at the weather and we would be flying into severe turbulence. I am a nurse, not a pilot, so I asked her to tell me what severe turbulence means, to talk to me like I was a five-year-old. She replied that we would be flying into weather that could cause her to lose control of the aircraft. I told her I wasn't going.

One of the directors came out of the office, asking why I was declining the flight. I said, "If she can't control the aircraft, then I'm not going." He was pissed, so I said, "I'll go if you go with me!" We then declined the flight. The weather was bad when that helicopter had crashed that one night. They flew right into a mountain.

Once, I had a patient, a gang member who had been shot in the heart. The radiology study revealed that the bullet came to rest on top of his pericardium, a fibrous sac that houses the heart. He went home. I was wondering how it was that killers would live, and these angels would die!

CHAPTER 28

I GOT A THANK YOU

Working as a float nurse was a ball. I learned a lot from running all over and working in multiple departments. The one thing I learned was that the nurses on the medical surgery floor were the hardest working nurses in the hospital. They often had upwards of five patients who needed baths, food, medication, toileting, diagnostics, more food, more toileting, more medication, etc. The nurses on AM shifts were especially busy, whereas the nurses on PM shifts had it made! ER nurses would flurry, then wait. ICU nurses could get busy, but they only had two patients at most. My ER skills proved handy on medical surgery: I could start IVs fast, hang medications, check blood sugars, and so on. The nurses loved me because I was around to make their days easier.

I would also help out in the ICU. While those Nurses went on their breaks, I would look after their patients. It was all good, but crazy things would happen. They always did!

I met Mr. Neary, a nice man and a retired military officer who had come in for gastrointestinal bleeding. I admitted him and scheduled him for scoping the next day. I was filling in for the nurse caring for Mr. Neary. They asked me to administer his medications. When I saw Mr. Neary, he asked for a Gatorade. I told him I would return in one moment. Upon my return, I saw him seize. I looked at his wife, who got out of the way, checked a pulse and found it was absent. I then started CPR. I saw my friend walk by and told him to bring in the crash cart. We hooked him up. Mr. Neary was in V-fib, so I shocked him. We had his airway, I pushed some epinephrine and shocked him again. We had vital signs! He coded three more times.

The doctor wanted to get him to the catheterization lab, which was 20 miles away. I don't know who set up the transfer, but a basic life support ambulance arrived. Clearly, they could not take him. I asked: "Is the catheterization lab his only hope?" The two doctors who were there said yes. I then offered to accompany the patient. We loaded him and went lights and sirens to the next hospital.

A week later, I got a phone call in the ICU. It was Mrs. Neary! She called to thank me and said her husband was doing fine. She wanted to send me a gift, but I informed her it was against hospital policy. She said the cardiologist told her that if it wasn't for "that nurse" doing what he did, Mr. Neary wouldn't be alive today! I thanked her and told her how happy I was to hear the news.

A month or so later, I saw Mr. Neary again on the medical surgical floor. I was walking past his room when I heard him yell, "Hey!" I went in the room. His sons were there, and they looked at me. Mr. Neary said, "I want to thank you for saving my life." I laughed and told him to thank Dr. Zoll, since he made the defibrillator! I was glad I went to work that day.

Across the hall, we had a patient who weighed about 400 pounds. He had been lying in a river of shit. This stuff was running out like the Mississippi! I turned him on his side using all the power from my quads to move him. The other nurses were cleaning him up. The patient was very appreciative and kept thanking us. He was on his cell phone with his wife. I'm sweating bullets trying to hold him in position while the other nurses are wiping his butt, and he is asking what kind of wine we like. I told him I liked red! He asked his wife to bring in a case. I couldn't wait. Months went by, and I never saw a bottle!

I was called to the ER to help with a patient. She was sick and unresponsive. The ER doctor was a horrible woman. She hated everyone, and I mean everyone, especially Hispanics and their children. Oftentimes, she would tell me to tell those families to go somewhere else. I would reply, "You tell them." It was always an awful experience having to work with her. I had witnessed her degrade a nursing supervisor so badly, the supervisor just broke down and quit nursing. That lady just could not go on, not one step further.

The doctor looked at the patient and said she would put in a central line but would not intubate. I was looking at the nurse and asking, "Are you kidding me?"

The nurse kept telling me, "Don't say anything." It was crazy; the patient clearly needed an airway. I helped out and then went back upstairs. After the patient's CT scan, she was admitted to the ICU. I went back down to help with the transfer. I could see the patient was declining and about to respiratory arrest while we were stuck in the elevator. The nurse I was with was freaking out and I was going off about the ER doctor. We got into the ICU and I called a code. Luckily, an intensive care doctor was there. He was about to intubate when the lady started vomiting coffee grounds, volcano-like. She was bleeding, and I was suctioning her airway with two Yankauer devices at the same time! The doctor got the tube, but the patient died.

Mr. Morry was admitted for progressive weakness related to his stomach cancer. During his stay, he received fluids and rest. The combination seemed to help quite a bit. He was visibly better. I was happy to see it, because I was almost certain it was his last admission. I didn't think that he would survive. One day, he had shit the bed and I was there to help clean him up. He was very weak. When I lifted him up and out of the bed, I held him close. I was basically hugging him. We got him clean and back in bed only to find that he had shit the bed again! I picked him up again, hugged him, and got him clean. That was that. The family was there, and they saw the care we gave to their husband and father.

Just before Mr. Morry was discharged, he yelled out for me from his room. He began to hand me an envelope with my name on it. I told him I could not accept a gift. He insisted, and my supervisor told me to take it. Mr. Morry gave me a certificate for a wonderful Italian dinner. My wife and I enjoyed it very much. It was his way of saying thank you!

Once, I was talking to a neighbor on my street as a woman approached me with her dog. She said I was her mother's nurse and thanked me for taking care of her mom and helping the family through a very difficult time. I had no recollection of it. She said she just wanted to thank me. That was nice. I found a card in my mailbox the next day.

CHAPTER 29

BACK TO THE ED

The ER was getting a bit busy, so the supervisor asked me to give the nurses lunch relief. An interesting set of dynamics had developed. My sense was that a few of the nurses harbored resentment towards me as a result of my having left. I thought it was a bit odd. Why would they care? What's more, they jacked up my schedule, which is why I left in the first place.

One nurse went to lunch and was late in returning. I was waiting for her when she called the department to tell me she was going to be even later. She was in line at a checkout stand at some clothing store. I really couldn't wait much longer; I had to give lunch breaks to other nurses.

Moments later, the paramedic radio alarmed. We were getting a two-year-old who'd had a seizure. When they arrived at the back door, the little boy was in his mother's arms. From there, they were directed to the crash room where I introduced myself to the mother and began assessing the patient.

I hooked up the patient to the cardiac monitor and noticed that the pulse oximeter was slow and did not correlate with the patient's cardiac activity. I walked over and further scrutinized the waveform as I looked at the little boy. My mind did not want to believe what my eyes were seeing. Actually, my mind did not want to believe what my eyes *weren't* seeing. The patient's chest was not moving—he had stopped breathing! I walked over to the crash cart and grabbed the Ambu bag (a self-inflating breathing bag) so I could ventilate the kid. Fortunately, a pediatrician just happened to be in the department. I nodded over at him and he walked over to the bed as I bagged the patient. The nurse who had returned late from lunch appeared and started screaming as we were working on the patient. I had to tell her, "No screaming, please leave." The doctor intubated her as I placed an IV and ordered a chest x-ray. I then took the patient to CT. When we returned from radiology, the doctor ordered mannitol to get fluid out of the patient's skull. He was stabilized and sent to the children's hospital.

As I walked out of the room, the clerk said to me, "There is an unresponsive kid in triage." I opened the door and the parents handed me their child. He was about six years old. He turned his head towards me, vomited, and lost consciousness. I had him in my arms as I checked the crash room. It was full, so I ran into an empty room, checked the patient's pulse, and started CPR. Luckily, the pediatrician was still there. We got the patient on a monitor. He was in pulseless V-tach, so we began CPR and defibrillated; I got an IV and gave epinephrine. We then checked his blood sugar, which was low, so we gave D25W. We continued CPR, defibrillated him, and he was intubated. He had equal breath sounds.

As a team, we had coded the patient for three hours. He was in and out of V-tach the whole time. Finally, when his rhythm stabilized, the transport team got him to the children's hospital. Later, I was told that both the patients had survived! I was so glad to hear the news. Again, I found myself so grateful for the time I had in the pediatrics ER so many years before. I often thought about the doctor who pushed me to be a PALS instructor and realized how much she had shaped my nursing career. As I was leaving, Lilly came up to me and asked me to wait. I stopped and turned. She was smiling and pressed herself up against me. I told her I had to go. I wanted none of that.

CHAPTER 30

NOBODY CARES?

At times, I would float into the ICU. I enjoyed the work, the nurses were cool and capable, and we generally had a good time. Still, I noticed there was one nurse who was a bit odd. Other nurses seemed to keep their distance from him. Nothing was ever said to me, so I never gave him much thought. I was always nice.

One day, a friend of mine was admitting a patient to the unit. As I was getting report, Mark, the odd duck, got in between us and started shouting at me, "Who do you think you are in here? This is my unit!" It was bizarre, but again I didn't give it too much thought. I figured he was just trying to be intimidating but I wasn't about to get shaken. One of the other nurses told me he did not like other men in the department. I knew a lot of nurses and have been around long enough to accept the dysfunction and pathology of the field. I was not bothered.

Dory was one of the nurses I really appreciated. We worked well together and always helped each other. We ended up getting into a contest over who would buy the other person a latte from the cafeteria. Yolie was another nurse in the ICU I admired. She had a lot of experience, which made it refreshing to work beside her. She truly cared for her patients and was a great role model for her fellow nurses.

I was taking care of a patient who'd suffered a stroke. I remember him as a very nice man. On this particular day, his family was coming by to see him. He had been in the unit for a few days and looked unkempt. I asked him if he would like to get cleaned up before his family arrived and he agreed. I bathed him, washed his hair, brushed his teeth, and gave him a fresh shave. He looked great, like a shiny copper penny!

His son arrived and couldn't believe his eyes. His dad looked great! He approached me and said he couldn't understand how his dad looked so presentable. He then asked me if I did it and I said yes. He wanted to know if his father asked me to do it and again I said yes. He was blown away. The little task I did was so worth it. That's nursing!

Now, all this had been done for the patient. I did my best to care for him and address the family's concerns. Everything was going well. I established their trust and confidence and then…a nursing supervisor came into the unit. She was a traveler. The hospital had to get someone right away because of the nurse we lost just a bit ago on account of that ER doctor. This supervisor was worthless. She spent all her time in the parking lot smoking. She finally came up to the ICU, knew nothing of my patient, and started screaming, "He needs to go!" The family lost it! I had to direct them to administration, since I could not do any damage control. It had been one of the most horrific experiences I had ever seen. They say nursing is a caring profession, but I was really beginning to wonder.

One day, Mark asked me to start an IV on his patient. I was happy to oblige, but I asked him if he had tried. Mark told me he couldn't start IVs. I mistakenly mentioned IVs were a basic nursing skill and questioned how he could really take care of an emergency if he didn't have IV skills. It was just a question, but Mark took offense at it. As I turned, he pushed me. Well, I reported the interaction and as a result we were both fired.

I couldn't believe it. I had to go home to my wife and kids and tell them I had lost my job. I guess the zero tolerance for violence in the workplace policy also applied to the victim.

CHAPTER 31

SOMETIMES IT'S WHO YOU KNOW

I was searching for a job everywhere. I needed something. I had been working in a small community and word travels fast. I scheduled an interview for an ER position. I figured I would be a shoo-in. I had a great conversation with my interviewer. She did ask if I was ever terminated; I found that odd. She told me to expect a call on Tuesday, but the call never came.

I was contacted by one of the ER doctors I knew. He wanted me in the ER where he was now the medical director. I showed up for the interview. It was good to see him. I had a nice talk with the manager, who offered me the position immediately. I was told to expect a call from HR on Monday. The call never came, and they never returned my calls.

I saw another job online. The place was looking for a charge nurse in their ER. I knew a couple of the pharmacists who worked there and had another friend who was a nursing supervisor there. I talked with them. They wanted me to come down and would put in a good word for me!

I met the manager. While the interview was fine, something felt off about him. His nose was big and a bit blue, and his face was flushed. I wondered if he had a problem with alcohol. I was also a bit skeptical because most charge nurses come up through the staff ranks. I couldn't help but wonder why they were searching on the outside. Anyway, he offered me the position and I took it. I was desperate after all.

Quite honestly, I had no idea what to expect. I figured I would keep my head down, work hard, and do my best to acclimate. Shortly after I'd started, the manager called me into the office. What he had to say was a bit unnerving. He spoke about the nursing staff, calling one nurse slow and another even slower. He went on to say that, yet another nurse should work in the gift shop. The next nurse on the list was described as a nymphomaniac, and the last was said to have ADD so badly, he wanted the guy out. The manager had nothing good to say about anyone. I wondered how long it would be before he started taking issue with me. The manager was demanding and wanted me to write everyone up. He said he expected a pile of reports on his desk. He also wanted me to keep an eye on the physicians!

I needed the job and I was willing to work, so I told him I would do my best as charge nurse. I also told him I wanted to make friends. He responded, "That is not why I'm hiring you!"

I said to him, "You know what's going to happen? They are all going to get upset with me and march in here. What then?"

He replied, "Fine, they can go. I'll fill this place with registry and travel nurses!" With that, I walked out, not knowing what the hell to expect. I was beginning to recognize that I really did not fit well in any of these small community hospitals.

A part of me hates to say it, but the manager was right. The ER was staffed with great people, but in no way were they ER nurses.

Some had been there between 15 and 25 years. Again, I was the new kid on the block. I was responsible for the ICU and what I saw there was, to put it mildly, horrifying.

CHAPTER 32

BACK IN CHARGE

I walked in for my first day with the sole intent to introduce myself, get to know the staff, and see how I could best help.

First, I met Allison. She seemed nice enough, though I immediately got the impression that she didn't want me anywhere near her patients. She had been in this little ER for 25 years. Her patients were her patients and the ER was her domain. She made clear that she had no use for me and it would be best for me to stay away. Of course, staying away was going to be a challenge on many levels. After all, I was hired to be the charge nurse, which carries a degree of responsibility and accountability. I also knew she lacked quite a bit of skill and knowledge. Accordingly, I was going to have to step in and help at times.

Darlene was another nurse I met. She was as nice as could be. I was greeted with a smile instantly. We worked well together. I was happy to work beside her. I was very lucky to build such a kind, warm friendship with her.

On another shift, I met the nymphomaniac. The manager could not have been more honest. When I first met her, I was charting on the computer. She slipped her hand over mine and whispered, "You can touch my mouse anytime." I'd been around long enough to know that saying nothing and walking away was my best option.

Later during the same shift, I was called to try to get an IV on a patient in the ICU. I walked up the stairway and saw the nymphomaniac nurse following me. She joined me in the ICU and stood beside me as I placed the IV line. She cut the tape and handed it to me, so I could secure the line. I knew she could be big trouble. As luck would have it, the nursing supervisor was present. She asked me what was going on. I told her I had no clue. That all of a sudden, this other nurse just appeared beside me. The supervisor shook her head and said the nymphomaniac was at it again. It was my first week and I could already tell the place was crazy.

The manager handed me a pile of forms that I was to complete. He was demanding that I detail extended patient wait times, poor medical decisions, and poor nursing interventions. He also told me he did not want the clerks triaging anyone! He wanted me to go after everyone, so I began to fill out the forms.

We had a patient who ended up with a seven-hour stay for a bruised arm. I wrote that one up. There was a stroke patient who had no labs drawn for two hours. I wrote that one up as well. I also wrote up an incident involving a clerk who went out to the waiting room, triaged a patient, and put him in a bed. Another patient suffered a head laceration and was left bleeding in a room. The floor was covered with his blood when I found him. He was cold, pale, and had experienced a significant drop in blood pressure. I started two 14-gauge IVs and opened up IV fluids. I then grabbed the doctor, who closed the wound. I guess his nurse was just watching him bleed. I had to write that one up, too.

Another nurse had a patient who was admitted for appendicitis. The operating room was coming to get the patient, and nothing had been done. There was no IV, no antibiotics were hung, there was an incomplete pre-op checklist, and the nurse had just left the department. He was hanging out in the radiology department without giving word to anyone! I had to write it up. Although I did write these incidents up, no corrective measures were taken. However, as I anticipated, I became an outcast.

The ICU was pathetic. I travelled up there one day and the nurse I was going to relieve asked me to hang some blood. I was happy to do so, but I looked at the paperwork to discover that the unit had been sitting out for two hours! The blood was no good, so I returned it to the lab.

I found another patient in bed breathing rapidly. I was concerned, so I listened to her lungs. She was wheezing up a storm. I checked her orders and saw that she had medication available. Even so, she had not received the bronchodilators for two days. It was crazy!

A different patient displayed a bizarre waveform on his pulse oximeter. The pulse rate on the pulse oximeter was half of what the ECG tracing showed. I checked his pulse, and sure enough his pulse was 36 but his heart was depolarizing at 72. I called his doctor and told him what I had found. I told him the electrical waveform activity of his heart revealed a rate of 72 per minute, however, the patient's actual heart beat was 36 per minute. His reply was, "I don't know what I'm going to do about that." Then he hung up the phone.

I was bewildered and not too sure what my role was going to be. The nurses and doctors were set in their ways, and I was not going to change anything. I thought I'd made a big mistake leaving the old county hospital. I loved working with so many brilliant, motivated doctors and nurses there. As much as I tried, I could never find another place like that. This place was a horror show by comparison. The patient care sucked, but I needed a job. After all, I had a family to support. Stuck between a rock and a hard place, I was determined to do my best to make it work.

It was a Saturday and I was going up to give breaks to the nurses in the ICU. One of the nurses seemed nice enough, but I could tell that her critical care skills were lacking. She had a female patient in respiratory distress. Evidently, the patient had a procedure and during sedation, aspirated gastric contents and had a bad pneumonia. The nurse left for break. I went to look at her patient, who was breathing about 60. She was awake and alert, but she was hurting. She was on both an oxygen mask and an oxygen cannula. She wanted some water to drink, so I removed the mask for her only to see her oxygen saturation plummet to 70 percent. I put the O2 back on, called respiratory therapy, and looked at her husband as he was sitting there. I think he had a sense of the severity of her illness. I later learned he was a paramedic and firefighter.

Sunday morning, I came into work, saw the nursing supervisor, and inquired about the lady in the ICU. I asked if she had been intubated. The supervisor didn't know. By noon, I went back to the unit to give lunch breaks. Another nurse was caring for the same patient. She ordered me not to touch the patient! The patient was in worse shape than she had been the previous day. To the best of my knowledge, she had been allowed to deteriorate in respiratory distress for at least three 12-hour shifts.

The nurse went to lunch I entered the room and looked at the patient. It was apparent that she was running out of steam. I was assessing her and after some deliberation, I contacted her doctor and told him I needed him here STAT. The patient needed intubation and ventilation immediately! I grabbed all the drugs we required, and sedation was administered. As the patient was tubed and vented, her oxygenation improved, and her heart rate began to normalize. I saw her husband near the elevator and told him things were looking up. He shook my hand, thanked me, then said, "I like the way you work." I walked away thinking I was happy I'd gone to work that day.

I saw the couple several times during the following days. The patient's husband and daughter would visit her often. She did get off the vent as her condition continued to improve. Ultimately, they all got to go home together.

I never got to a point of understanding how some nurses could be so territorial when their actions impacted patient outcomes so negatively. What I did begin to realize was that the territorial attitude was inversely proportional to competence. The bigger the attitude, generally the less competent the nurse.

The days, weeks, months passed. Very little changed. One day, a three-month-old baby came in vomiting with a fever. I knew he needed admission and transfer. His mother brought him in but didn't want anything done and left. Two days later, the baby returned with the same complaints. I was trying my best to do the work up, but the doctor entered and said, "We are not going to do anything for the baby." I looked at him and the mother, thinking both of them were nuts. I had seen a lot of sick kids and this was one of them. The shift was coming to an end, and I was going home.

Two days later, the same child arrives by ambulance. He was weak, mottled, and his circulatory blood volume was depleted. Upon his arrival, he was sent to nurse Allison. Now, this was the first time Allison ever asked for help or would allow me to stand over her patient! I understood why. She was clearly out of her comfort zone. I stepped in to help. The patient had no veins, so I placed an IO needle into his tibia. To the mother, I explained how and why we were doing what we were doing. The line was placed and flushed with 30 ml of normal saline. It was working fine.

Allison was to administer another 150 ml of normal saline. After a bit, she called me back to look at the patient's leg. It was largely swollen. I soon discovered that Allison's actions had dislodged the needle, which she neglected to assess until all the fluid was in the patient's soft tissue. His mother was hysterical. We got the child transferred, but I never found out if he survived. The truth is that I would have loved to have worked on him four days earlier, but I'm just a nurse.

I remember working with Dr. Faust, who was a real piece of work. I don't know how to describe him other than to say that I couldn't believe he graduated from medical school. I walked in one day to find him in front of his computer, on Facebook! I think he wanted to be a model or something. The guy was a trip.

Anyway, I relieved a nurse caring for a man who was short of breath. I walked in to see his respiratory rate at 60, his O2 sat on a mask at 60 percent, and his blood pressure at 60! I began to move him into the crash room and told Dr. Faust I needed him. But he was still on Facebook. I guess he didn't want to get off the computer!

I had the patient hooked up on the cardiac monitor and oxygen in the crash room and told the doctor that the patient's blood pressure was very low. I wanted to start another IV and hang Levophed, a vasopressor medication. The doctor's back was still towards me as he told me he was going to put in a big central line. I set everything up for the line and saw the patient deteriorating further. I told the doctor that the patient couldn't breathe!

The doctor put his hand up, as if to silence me! Now, I turned toward the patient's wife and locked eyes with her as I yelled, "Dr. Faust, I'm telling you the man cannot breathe!" He finally got up from that computer after 40 minutes of my pushing him to see the patient. Immediately, he scrambled to intubate him. During the intubation, the patient had a cardiac arrest. I started CPR and gave epinephrine. The patient regained his pulse, so I finally got to hang the vasopressor. Now intubated and stabilized, we moved him to the ICU.

The patient's wife looked at me later and said she could not believe the doctor refused to get off his computer and kept ignoring me. I had no response. After all, I was just a nurse. As we brought the patient upstairs, I was charged with giving report on the patient to the ICU nurse who was now pissed she was getting the patient. All I could do was hope for the best for this guy. Yes, he was sick, but it could very well be this hospital that killed him.

Sometimes I just don't get nurses. I wondered how they could get so upset about receiving patients. I would wonder if gas station attendants got upset when people came in for a fill-up. That's about as much sense it made to me. Sick people end up in hospitals and in ICUs, cars low on fuel go to gas stations, right?

I recalled a time about 25 years earlier when I was heading into the pediatric ER. As I walked through the main ER waiting room, I could detect the unmistakable smell of shit. I worked a PM shift and stayed to work overtime. By one in the morning, that stench was wafting into the pediatric ER nurse's station. I headed back to the big waiting room to see if I could locate the origin of the smell. What I found was a little old lady who was wheelchair bound. It was her. I asked if she'd like to get cleaned up, and she nodded affirmatively. I wondered how this situation was allowed to continue over the day and into the night shift (those waits were often 12 plus hours). After all, six nurses, three clerks, and three shift supervisors worked right beside this person through the course of that entire time.

I wheeled the lady back to the newly remodeled psych ER that had a shower, but the psych nurse who met us refused to allow me to clean the patient, stating the patient was not a psych patient!

Well, I got on the phone with the director of nursing that moment. I woke her up and detailed the account. She called me back in less than five minutes, and I was able to get the lady a nice warm shower and some clean clothes. I loved being a nurse, but it ain't easy sometimes.

CHAPTER 33

TIMING IS EVERYTHING

My son's girlfriend had a cold and ended up giving it to him. Somehow, both my wife and I also got the cold. It was a Thursday night and we'd gone to bed early, something we both never do. We woke rested the next morning, and my bride made me a fried egg sandwich. I packed my lunch and I was off to work.

Later that afternoon, she texted saying she had a constant cough. What was I supposed to do? I was at work and I had the cold, too. I was thinking, "You've got to be kidding me." Hours later, our son texts me saying, "Mom can't breathe, and she won't let me take her to the hospital." Now, I know he can be a bit of a drama queen, so I wasn't getting shaken up. Besides, I'm an ER nurse and we don't go to the hospital unless we are dying!

He texted again and told me her temperature was 102.2°F. I instructed him to bring her to the hospital near our house. Work was slow, so I was able to leave early and meet them there. When I got to the hospital, they were yet to arrive. Finally, they pulled up and my wife got out of the car. She was hunched over and breathing like a locomotive. I was wondering what the hell was going on. We brought her back to a bed immediately.

She looked pasty. Her cardiac monitor showed a tachycardia in the 130s, her O2 sat was in the low 80s, and she was breathing about 50. Her nurse came up to me, and the first thing he told me was that he was a flight nurse! He had a bit of an ego, which was made worse by the fact that I was in my scrubs. It was clear he needed to establish his authority. I was trying to be cool and asked which company he worked for. It turns out that it was the same company I'd worked with in years past. I told him that I spent some time there and asked if he knew some of my old friends. I was hoping we could find some common ground—that never happened.

I asked the flight nurse if we could bump up my wife's O2 since she was breathing at 50. He responded, "No, she's breathing at 24. Look at the monitor." Now anyone worth their salt knows to look at the patient, not the monitor. I clearly wasn't getting anywhere. My wife received some IV fluid, IV antibiotics, and a breathing treatment to open her airways a bit, but I could tell nothing was improving. She began to complain of tightness in her abdomen, so the doctor gave her a touch of Dilaudid, a narcotic analgesic.

The flight nurse was not paying much attention to my wife. I could tell he wasn't concerned about her, plus we never established warm and fuzzies. The blood pressure recycled and read 60. I then checked her radial pulse and it was absent. I alerted the nurse immediately. He turned to me and said he didn't believe it! It was a throwback to the pediatrician who didn't believe me when I told him about the patient with a whited-out lung. He didn't believe it either, and the patient died! I suggested that we start a vasopressor and bump up her O2. In response, he said he didn't want to bring out the "big guns." What I wanted to say was, "Hey asshole, she's tachypneic, tachycardic, hypoxic, and hypotensive! A half milligram of Dilaudid did not do this to her!" Instead, I grabbed an O2 mask off the wall to place over her.

At that moment, the doctor returned and in his all-powerful voice said, "Look, you're a family member now. Just sit down and chill out!" I was looking down at my wife and thinking, "27 years of critical care and ER nursing and there is nothing I can do for you. I have to sit here and watch this happen. I can't start another IV, I can't give you oxygen, or start a vasopressor. With everything I've learned and all the skills I've gained, I can't do anything. If I go off on these guys, they'll call security and I need them to focus on you." With that, I stepped out to the ambulance entrance to tell my boys their mom was sick and needed to be admitted.

For some reason, I didn't stay there long. I walked back into the room to find the physician attempting to intubate my wife. It was obvious that he was struggling. I told him to get a smaller tube! I then looked at the monitor and saw her flatline! I screamed, "Check a pulse, get some epinephrine and some atropine. Start CPR, now people, now!" Her care providers neglected to watch her vital signs during the intubation! They did not notice the bradycardia and the drop in her O2 saturation. They stared at my wife's mouth as the doctor was wrestling to get the tube in.

I watched the ER technician doing CPR. It was weak and slow. As I watched him, I heard my wife's voice in my head saying, "You're not going to just stand there and watch this, are you?" With that, I ripped off my jacket, jumped into the flight nurse's face, and said "I'm doing CPR!" My compressions were fast and hard. I was doing CPR like my life depended on it and it did. I remember screaming, "Come on baby, come on!" In my head I was thinking, "It's not going to happen like this, not tonight. Our story isn't ending like this." I was envisioning the code calling. I could see myself stepping off the CPR stool, walking down the hall, and telling my boys that their mother had died! I was not going to let it happen! I kept screaming and compressing, calling out for epinephrine. The doctor finally got the tube. My wife had regained her pulse!

After the intubation, everyone left. I was there by myself with my wife on the ventilator. I was wondering where the hell everyone went. Her tube was filling up with bloody, foamy sputum. I was suctioning her mouth and suctioning her tube to keep her airway clear. I was so happy I had all the skills to manage her airway!

A few hours later, she was admitted to the ICU and I was accompanying the transfer. Leaving the ER, I could not feel a pulse, so I informed the flight nurse. He responded, "She just had a blood pressure!" It was two in the morning. I had been up for 21 hours and coded my wife twice. I looked at him and thought, "I'm tired of arguing with you." I figured if she was dead, she was dead. We proceeded to the elevator.

Arriving in the ICU, I screamed for a Doppler (a device revealing sound waves created by blood coursing through the artery allowing me to measure her blood pressure). My wife's blood pressure was 50. I stayed beside her. A nurse walked in and said, "Hey, you were my ACLS instructor!" I asked if she passed!

I knew these nurses wanted my wife to survive. I was one of them! They wanted her to live for me!

By morning, my wife's blood pressure was supported by Levophed, vasopressin, Neo-Synephrine, and dobutamine. She was vented on 100 percent oxygen, her blood pressure was 70, her O2 saturation was 70, and her pupils remained fixed and dilated. I called my boss, apologized for waking him, and told him I wouldn't be at work for a while, as my wife had a cardiac arrest. I went home to shower, but I couldn't sleep.

I returned to meet the new doctor. He was another intensivist. I could tell he was sharp as a tack. We had a good conversation, and I was reassured by the fact that he was doing his best. I was feeling hopeless, but I knew that he was trying to save her and comfort me. I looked at him and said, "Come on, she's in multi-organ dysfunction."

He replied, "Yes, but she's not in multi-organ failure." With that, he gave me hope.

The time had come for a shift change. I was about to meet one of the best nurses I'd ever know. Her name was Kathy, and she was an angel. She was just what my family and I needed!

She introduced herself, assessed her patient, and checked all the IV lines. She was doing her job, and she was doing it well. We talked a bit and she was feeling me out. She asked if it was true that I'd performed CPR on my wife in the ER. I responded yes. You could tell there weren't many nurses in the ICU who were proud of their ER. Inside, I chuckled because I never knew an ICU nurse who thought much of an ER nurse. It's all about hierarchy. Kathy did a great job. She gave excellent nursing care to my wife and our family. She kept my wife clean and groomed, kept her alive, and always gave us hope. She was just what we needed.

After my wife had spent a week on the ventilator, the doctor decided it was time to extubate her, to take out the breathing tube. I was there beside him when he pulled the tube. Previously, the ventilator weaning trials were okay, but once the tube was pulled she only lasted 10 minutes. I grabbed the doctor and said, "This is where we were last week." He set up to intubate.

A nurse pushed some Propofol to get her back to sleep, all while I was bagging (ventilating her with the Ambu bag). She was reintubated, sedated, and placed back on the ventilator.

I could tell the doctor was bummed. He said to me, "Maybe in a few more days."

I said, "How about another week." He just looked at me.

It was hard to endure. I never thought I would be bagging my wife. Last week, I was doing CPR. This was too much. It had been a week since I heard her voice or felt her touch. My cousin Tommy called and asked me what was going on. I gave him the blow-by-blow. Tommy and I always had a close relationship. I loved him as much as you could love anyone. He was more than a brother. We shared our lives together since we were kids. I remember the one thing he turned me onto was a movie titled *The Big Lebowski*. We had each seen this film over 20 times.

When Tommy asked me about why things were so bad in the ER I told him, in my best Walter Sobchak, "Cause they're a bunch of fucking amateurs!" We had a good laugh at that! Tommy bought a plane ticket and was out in two days. It was a very good thing because, to quote the movie, "Darkness washed over the dude, darker than a black steer's tookus on a moonless prairie night. There was no bottom."

My bride was holding her own on the ventilator and the vasopressors. I was very grateful for the invention of electricity and glad the hospital was paying their electric bill. Kathy returned, and I was really happy to see her. Things weren't getting better, but they weren't getting worse until Kathy told me she would be going on vacation. How could she leave us at a time like this?

CHAPTER 34

WHAT A DIFFERENCE A WEEK MAKES

The days dragged on. As each one passed, it became more and more difficult for all of us. I watched my wife on the ventilator, she was out of touch. Her electrolytes were out of whack and her heart rhythm was all over the place. It looked like certain doom at times. Her monitor alarms were going off constantly.

A new nurse named Norma arrived. She appeared very old and feeble. I sat there in the room thinking, "You've got to be kidding me." My wife's right subclavian line was going to be discontinued, as they placed a new IV line in her left arm. This now meant that all her IV lines needed to be changed over. I could see Norma was a bit overwhelmed, so I offered to help her. She replied that it was against the hospital policy.

I sat in a chair at the foot of the bed while she was trying to figure out what to do. She said, "At first, well I'll just turn off all the pumps and move them." I was so glad I was there. I told her that she could not do that. There were sedatives and vasopressors infusing that couldn't be turned off without the patient (my wife) crashing. She then tried to move the pumps, which required her to lift them over the O2 supply lines that fed the ventilator. Needless to say, that was a challenge for her. I watched as she kept pushing the ventilator out the door with her big butt. Suddenly, I jumped out of the chair and grabbed my wife's endotracheal tube! Nurse Norma unknowingly almost extubated my wife! At that point, I did not hesitate to intervene. I told her that I'd transferred patients on a ventilator with arterial lines, a transvenous pacer, and four IVs in a helicopter. I'm doing this! I anticipated her objection and said I didn't care about hospital policy or the Board of Registered Nursing. I was moving the pumps. She got out of my way. I changed everything over without incident and then told her to go ahead. Though I helped her discontinue the subclavian line, she then contaminated it. As a result, it was of no use to send the tip to the lab to be cultured.

The week progressed, and it was up and down. The ventilator weaning trials seemed favorable. I thought, "Maybe, just maybe she could get off the vent!" Kathy was back! The doctor had come into the room to talk to me about a few things. I knew what he wanted to address. One was a possible tracheostomy tube if she couldn't get off the ventilator, and the other was a feeding tube. Nutritional needs had to be addressed, I understood. I asked the doctor if we could wait a bit on the feeding tube. He was perplexed and asked why. I told him I liked my wife a little skinnier. He couldn't hold back the laughter. Kathy gave me a swift kick in the butt, and she kicked me hard!

The time had come. It was either off the ventilator or to the OR for a tracheostomy. I couldn't take much more, so I left the hospital and went for a walk. I didn't want to return.

That afternoon, I did go back hesitantly. I walked up to the ICU door that had some film torn away off the privacy glass. I peered through the hole, and I could see into my wife's room. The ventilator was off! That could only mean one of two things: she was either alive and breathing on her own or she wasn't. I rang the bell. Kathy opened the door. I saw that my wife was awake and sitting up. Sunlight filled her room. I felt like Rocky Balboa, "Yo, Adrian! We did it!" I couldn't hold back my tears.

CHAPTER 35

EXIT STAGE RIGHT

My wife was soon discharged home, and everyone was elated. I went back to work. I was still pretty numb from the previous 28 days of living on the edge.

As soon as I got into the department, the manager came to see me. We walked into the office. It seemed we had a problem, which apparently needed addressing upon my immediate return. I guess in my absence a number of the staff had voiced numerous complaints about me. Exactly what I had predicted months ago had come to pass.

The manager put me in a position to do his work and clean up the staff. Against my better judgement, I did what he asked because I needed a job. Now, I was taking the heat. I reminded him of my prediction that the staff eventually would band against me, but he would have none of it. It was all my fault and came down to my lack of adequate communication skills. I rebutted that I was a grown man, a professional, and that I did know how to communicate. I told him I really did not know how to move forward from here. All he said was he'd give me two weeks to figure it out. I left the office and went to work.

The next day, he called me into his office again. He confronted me again, the second time in 24 hours. I couldn't believe it. He repeated everything we spoke about the day before. He then said, "You look like a bull with his balls cut off. You look like a dog with his tail between his legs!" I just sat in the chair and took a deep breath. He just sat there talking shit.

The next weekend, I was teaching an ACLS class. I saw an old friend, Jenny. I knew her from about 20 years before. She was a sight for sore eyes! We had a great visit. I was more interested in her than whether she knew the current treatment protocols. Turned out she was managing an ER and an ICU at another hospital. The place just so happened to be closer to me and paid more. I asked her if they needed anyone. We made an appointment to meet again on Monday. Well, we met, had coffee, caught up on the last 20 years, and I got the job! I would be bouncing between the ICU and the ER in addition to taking some call time for special procedures. I couldn't have been happier.

I had to do a couple things before I gave notice. First, I wanted to apologize to my fellow nurses and somehow explain to them that the person they knew wasn't me. I wanted them to know that against my better judgement, in a moment of weakness, I acted how the manager had wanted. They were all very kind and quickly forgave me, but that wasn't enough for me. Armed with a voice recorder, I walked into the manager's office. I baited him by saying, "You know, you told me to go after slow and slower and ride the nympho's ass. Those were your words! You told me to go after the tech. You said you'd fire them and hire registry. Now I'm in the middle!" Well, he took the bait and rambled for 40 minutes on record. I got what I wanted and shared the conversation with the staff. I was cleared, and they got the picture!

I gave my two weeks' notice and couldn't have been happier to be getting out of there. My last day was a Friday. The manager asked if I could at least work the weekend. I had to laugh because there was no way. When I arrived on my last Friday shift, he met me at the time clock. We went to his office and he said he needed my ID badge. I gave it to him without hesitation, and he handed me my last check. He then said, "Now, I will escort you out of the building." I looked at him like he was a clown. I was the one who quit, and he was playing it as if I was some kind of threat or discipline case.

He was determined to march me out the front door, but as we walked down the hall I saw a side exit by radiology. I made an abrupt right and went out the exit. Looking back at him, all I could think was, "So long, sucker!" Now I was going to be working beside an old friend, closer to home, and making more money. I couldn't wait to get started. Everything was going to be better!

CHAPTER 36

OUTTA THE PAN, INTO THE FIRE

As time went on, I continued to be haunted by the words of my old friend. He warned me that I'd never find an ER like the one at old county. Everywhere I turned, it became truer. As I began my new job, I walked into the ER to introduce myself. I first met an ER technician, who seemed nice enough. There were two other nurses who looked pretty young. The guy seemed all right and easily approachable. The girl, however, struck me with a vibe immediately. She made no effort to raise her head up from her iPad, where she was engaged in a game of Candy Crush Saga. She just kept herself perched on a chair in the corner and never looked up.

That morning, the ER technician kept my attention. He showed me the entire department: where everything was kept and where to find more stock. He was doing what a nurse should have been doing. I was very impressed.

The hospital was very interesting. It was located on the outskirts of town, in the middle of an old hippie community. I was reminded of a flight I had taken to transport a patient back to the city. The place was way up north. Upon arriving into the ICU, I found one patient, alone on a ventilator, with no staff in sight. Suddenly, a nurse appeared from the outdoor patio with hair down to the middle of his back. He had just finished a few tokes off his Bob Marley joint. It would have been laughable had there not been a poor patient with a tube in his throat on a ventilator while his nurse was outside partying. It was a different culture.

The paramedic radio alarmed. We were alerted that they were on their way with an unresponsive child. I heard the doctor say, "Don't bring her here!" I never heard that from an ER doctor before. The patient arrived. She was a young girl, about three or four years old. When she arrived, she was unresponsive but warm and dry. Her pulse was good, and she was breathing fine. Her blood sugar was normal, and there was no trauma. Things didn't add up. It was clear that the staff was not pediatric ER trained, so I stepped in and placed the patient on a monitor. I got an IV, drew her blood, then placed a urinary catheter.

I watched the patient as the urine toxicology screen came back positive for cannabis! Well, the parents arrived, and it was determined that their baby got into their stash of marijuana butter! You can't write this stuff! The baby did fine. She probably would have liked a Snickers bar!

I got into a conversation with one of the nurses. We talked about ER nursing, and he had asked where I started. I gave him the lowdown on my experience over the years. Soon after the shift was over, I arrived home and my phone rang. It was Jenny. She was asking how my day went, and I said, "Fine." She said she needed to talk to me and told me she got some feedback. I was thinking, "Already? After one 12-hour shift?" I was told that the video game nurse had approached Jenny and expressed that she was not pleased with me. Evidently, she said that I was trying to sell myself as a nurse! I was blown away. I said to Jenny, "I don't even know what that means!" I don't think she did either.

Jenny knew me from way back, so she left it alone, saying "Just be yourself!" I knew from then on that the nurse with the video game was going to be trouble. I kept my distance as best I could. I wasn't too concerned about her because there was no way she'd get to me through Jenny.

I walked into the department one day to find Jenny. She asked me to take a look at a patient in bed five. I said, "Sure." I thought it was a bit odd, since there were two nurses in the department. Why would she ask me to peer in? Anyhow, I looked at the patient. He was pale. The respiratory therapist was trying to get a blood gas from his radial artery, though it clearly wasn't happening. I checked the patient's blood pressure and found that it was 40! Of course, he couldn't get a radial artery blood gas—the patient had no radial pulse! I noticed the patient had a small 20 g IV in his hand. The IV fluid was on a pump, which meant it would take an hour to get 1,000 ml of saline in him. So, I shoved in two 14 g IVs and opened up fluids with a pressure bag. I then grabbed the doctor and started a vasopressor. We got the patient into the ICU. I couldn't help noticing that while all this was going on, his nurse, the younger guy, was sitting across from the room at the nurse's station watching skateboarding videos on YouTube! Again, you just can't write this stuff!

I'm glad Jenny asked me to look in on the patient. The patient's wife was in the room during my flurry. She thanked me and said she liked the way I worked! The man ultimately survived and left the hospital doing very well. I was happy to see that.

Sometimes the hallways in the hospital smelled of marijuana. I wasn't sure if it was the staff or the patients! I walked into the ICU one day to find a patient smoking a joint in bed three. I had to take her lighter away, lest we get blown up with all the oxygen flowing!

It can be said that ICU nurses are the same everywhere. As I've previously mentioned, I discovered that attitude and competence are often inversely proportional! I went into the ICU to give a lunch break and met Elaine. As she was giving me report, I was ordered not to touch her patient! I was left wondering how she could ever say such a thing since in her absence I would be assuming responsibility for the patient's care—but "whatever." The doctor came in and made some changes. I titrated the IV drips, since the patient was on a ventilator and placed him on the ETCO2 monitor to keep track of his carbon dioxide levels. It also allowed me to monitor respiratory patterns. When Elaine returned from lunch, she was pissed! She ordered me to take the guy off the CO2 monitor.

I was breaking the other nurse when I noticed Elaine's patient was experiencing runs of V-tach. She didn't know what to do and was calling the doctor for orders. I mentioned that the doctor did write orders for an amiodarone infusion to treat the ventricular ectopy, but she ignored me and the orders that were in place. Finally, she got the confirmation she needed and began the infusion. I could see she was struggling to figure out the drip rate. As a result, she was flooding the medication into the patient too rapidly. I told her the rate should be 600 ml/hour, and she asked me how I determined the infusion rate. I answered, but she wasn't satisfied. She called the pharmacy, and the rate they gave her was the same as mine. The problem now was that the medication had been completely infused by the time she was about to make the rate correction. Consequently, the patient's heart rate slowed down so much that he required the use of a transcutaneous pacemaker. She had no clue about its function! I was happy to help her hook the patient up to the monitor and place the pads on his chest. I then informed her how to adjust the heart rate and the milliamperage, so we could capture the heart and keep it beating at the prescribed rate. The process was beyond her, but I was there to help. Unbeknown to me, she kept messing with the milliamperage. When the cardiologist arrived, he looked at her and said, "You know, you don't have capture!" I was working in a circus of clowns!

I was working in triage one day and met a clerk. He was a nice guy and he happened to be a surf rat, so I instantly liked him. We spent time swapping our amazing surf stories. He was sharp, and you could tell he had all kinds of potential. We would do our time, tell stories, and laugh. It was good. One day, he asked me what was up with me and nurse video game. Evidently, she told him that she sat me down, had a talk with me, and put me in my place! I was laughing so hard! First, I responded, "Do I look like the kind of guy who would be put in my place by her!" I then told him that he should be wary of a person who would make up an interaction. I informed him that the nurse and I never had the encounter she described to him. What I began to recognize in this ER was a culture of apathy and hate. There were nurses there (not all) who really did not care.

There was one nurse with jet black hair and sunken eyes. She would often be outside and smoked constantly. I would keep my distance from her as best I could because her vibe was so toxic. One day, she had a patient in alcohol withdrawal. She put him in a room and closed the door. The patient was sick, shaking, and had soiled himself completely. He was a hopeless mess, and she could not have cared less. I entered his room, cleaned the man, and warmed him up. Then, I summoned the doctor. The patient quickly improved with IV fluids and Ativan.

Moments later the clerk out front asked me to look at a patient in the waiting room. I guess nurse video game got the patient out of a car only to sit her in a chair in the waiting room and walk away. I found the patient barely responsive. She was ice cold, dirty, and her hands had been eaten by her cats. I called for Mary, an absolute angel of a nurse. Together, we moved the patient into a bed, warmed her with a heating blanket, bathed her, began fluid resuscitation, and dressed her wounds. It was heartbreaking! What kind of nurse would walk away from someone so ill? How did this patient get so neglected?

Time went on, and Jenny planned to move on to another job with more pay and better benefits. I was happy for her but sad to see her go. I was also a bit concerned that I was losing my only protection. Our new manager was Nancy. My first impression was that she was wired a bit tightly. Interestingly, she also seemed a bit more clueless about managing the place. I could tell her ability would be lacking. I just had a gut feeling.

Sure enough, I was called into her office two weeks later. She directed me to have a sit down with nurse video game! I began to tell her that I was not comfortable with it. I explained that the nurse had been creating discord for me since my first day. I relayed all that I had experienced of her as well as things that she had been saying about me from other staff. Nancy retorted that I was only reciting hearsay!

I explained that I didn't trust nurse video game, I did not want to be alone with her, and that I'd grown tired of taking her shit for the past year. Nancy began yelling at me. I recognized that the manager was not about to give me any validity but believed everything this other nurse had to say. I envisioned working beside nurse video game and I just couldn't do it! I told Nancy I wasn't feeling good about it at all. She then slammed her hand down on her desk and ordered me out of her office! I then told her I wasn't feeling too well and would be going home. The moment I got home, I received a call from Human Resources. I had an appointment the next day.

I walked in the next day to find Nancy with the director of nursing and an HR representative. Nancy began by laying into me about refusing to meet with the nurse. She then talked about how I began yelling and swearing and said that I frightened her. She wanted me suspended! Now, it was my turn!

I told them my side about nurse video and relayed that Nancy would not hear my side or recognize my apprehension about being alone with the nurse. I then shared my experience of Nancy yelling and slamming her hand on the desk. I even offered to demonstrate her behavior. I admitted to saying the word "shit," which she said was offensive! To that, I apologized and said I would never use the word shit again! I then asked Nancy why she was frightened of me. Did she think I was going to murder her?

Nancy then accused me of treating some nurses differently than others. I wanted to laugh! I responded, "You know there are some people you just groove with. They make your days fun." I acknowledged that I did treat some other nurses differently, but in the end, I respected people as people, but I may not respect them as nurses. I told her why: "While they are leaving a patient cold, lying in shit, and withdrawing from alcohol, I don't close the door and neglect him. I care for him. When another patient is unresponsive, filthy, and her hands are eaten away by cats, I don't stick her in a corner and walk away. I care for her! But those are your nurses, and they are your problem!" The manager looked at me and said it was my problem. I responded, "They are your nurses!"

As the meeting came to an end, the director clearly saw truth. She said there was no reason to suspend me and asked if I would meet with nurse video game the next day in HR, to which I agreed.

The next day, I walked into HR. Nurse video game stepped in and before I could say anything, she immediately said, "I'm so sorry it had to come to this!" She went on to say, "I cannot imagine how hard it is to do your job, to float all over the hospital, breaking everyone, and running from here to there constantly."

I just looked at her and said, "It's okay, we just had a breakdown in communication." With that, we hugged, and the meeting was over. As she was excused, I was asked to remain.

The HR representative asked me what the hell was going on. I asked her if she wanted the truth and she said yes. I basically told her that the ER was made up of cliques. The nurses were not very good, and the culture bred resentment for patients. I was asked my feelings of the manager, to which I replied, "I am very apprehensive around her. The fact she took our interaction and escalated it to this point concerns me. I do not feel safe around her."

The representative told me not to worry. She said that management was held to the same standards as every other employee. She insinuated that the manager had an issue with men and a history of physical abuse. She then smiled and said, "Just go to work. Do what you do and be yourself." That was nice. I came to find the hospital's finances were unstable. Closing was in the wind, so I began a new job search.

CHAPTER 37

SOME THINGS NEVER CHANGE

As luck would have it, I landed another job immediately. I was back doing critical care transports, which meant 24-hour shifts.

It didn't take too long to realize that the EMT staff never changed. I found these young kids to be immature. Most couldn't focus, so I had to not only look out for the patient, but also watch my staff to ensure they wouldn't make anything worse. However, some of the staff were really good. They knew their stuff, conducted themselves professionally. and made the job easier.

Still, I realized I was getting older. When some of the EMTs were driving too fast for conditions, I often thought we would all die in a crash. I found myself attempting to remind them that the patient was already in a hospital. Our transport was not a 911 emergency. When moving the patient, IV lines would get so tangled that I spent a lot of time getting them straight. I failed in my attempt to educate them about the importance of keeping lines free. They would not or could not grasp it. One day, as I was bouncing around, trying to push a medication that would be compatible with the infusion, I looked at my EMT and asked, "How many times have I stressed the importance of keeping IVs straight?"

He responded, "I don't know, six or seven?"

Other days became unbearable. I'd be assessing a patient at the bedside only to be squirted by saline flushes from another EMT. Apparently, it was fun for them to mess with the nurse. One of the other nurses came into the quarters in tears. I guess the lack of sleep, the responsibility of the job, and the constant needling from the EMTs finally got to him. He was a Native American and they kept calling him "chief." When he asked them to help and do their jobs, they often responded with "how?" He couldn't take it anymore.

I was sleeping when one of the kids kicked my door. He did it not once, but 15 times as hard as he could. He entered my room and told me to get up because he wanted to go to the store and buy some food. It was all I could take not to get up out of the bed and smash his head against a wall! Another time, the same kid drove away in the ambulance after I dropped a patient off in an ICU. I had to walk a half mile to get back in the rig. They had a great laugh!

The straw for me was when the EMT kept driving over the lane divider discs for miles, which was causing a loud vibration in the back where I sat. It was mind-numbing. I finally had to go to the management. I just didn't get how these kids could behave towards a person 30 years their elder, and a medical professional at that.

The nature of the work was challenging. We would often transport the sickest patients out of the hospitals that couldn't care for them to other hospitals that were better equipped. We had to keep the patient alive while doing so. The biggest changes I noticed on my return to transport nursing over the years was the overall decline in medical and nursing care. Back in the day, I would load the patient up and get on the road, but those days were gone! Now, it seemed almost every patient that I was called to transfer required stabilization. I found them in bad condition in the hospital while they were waiting for me to get them out. It seemed as if nobody cared!

We rolled into the ambulance bay of one of the hospitals. As I was helping the driver back the rig up, I was met by a respiratory therapist saying we'd better hurry up because the patient needed to be transferred. I was like, "Dude, we aren't even parked yet. If the patient is that bad off, you have a building with 100 doctors and at least 200 nurses. This isn't my emergency."

The crew and I got up to the floor to see the patient pale and hooked up to a BiPAP machine that was supposed to help her breathe. Nonetheless, she was deteriorating. The respiratory therapist gave me her latest blood gas result. I asked the patient if she was getting tired and she nodded affirmatively. I then told the respiratory therapist, "I'm not going anywhere until a physician is here at her bedside to reevaluate the patient."

A few moments later, an anesthesiologist showed up. He was a bit condescending and asked what the issue was. I gave him the blood gas results, told him the patient was tired, and said, "I can tube her en route, but I think it's safer to manage her airway here." He looked at me, then left to get his tools and meds. He returned and intubated the patient. I placed her on my monitor and ventilator when I noticed her blood pressure drop to 40. We gave IV fluids, and I started a Levophed drip that would elevate her blood pressure by vasoconstriction. The patient's cardiologist appeared moments later, she was going ballistic! She wanted dobutamine, which we didn't have. Their pharmacy had to mix it, and they needed an order. The problem was that the patient had no blood pressure now! I was looking at the cardiologist thinking, "You're the one who let the patient get like this!" I titrated the medication and packaged the patient for transfer.

The anesthesiologist was watching everything. He approached me and said, "Yeah, tubing her was the right call!"

I was like, "You think?"

Then he turned to me and said something very profound, "I think the best thing was you guys showing up!" I just smiled. We arrived at the receiving facility. The nurse who received the patient report began reprimanding me for not labeling the bag of Levophed.

We were transferring a young man to the city for surgery. I spoke to the nurse who had been caring for him over the last 12 hours, then went in to introduce myself. I could see the patient was in a lot of pain. I took his vital signs and found he had an elevated temperature and rapid heart rate. I went to the nurse's station and asked to speak with his doctor, who was a surgeon I knew from way back. I informed him of his patient's condition, and he told me I should drive faster! I said okay and hung up. A few moments later, the surgeon called me back and ordered more IV fluids. About this time, the nursing supervisor approached me with a scowl on her face. I was guessing she heard I was talking to the patient's doctor. She asked if there was a problem and I replied, "No, I found the patient febrile and spoke to his doctor." In response, she entered the patient's room and retook his vitals. She was obviously pissed about the situation. I guess it sucks when a nurse comes in off the street, assesses the situation, and takes charge! The resident showed up and called the receiving facility. I was then handed a couple doses of IV antibiotics to infuse en route.

My crew said, "Wow, you are a patient advocate!" I only thought I was doing my job. In doing so, I was saving the patient close to eight hours of down time waiting for the right medication to combat his infection.

A different call sent me to a hospital where I worked a while back. I walked into the ER and the manager came marching in at the same time. When he saw me, he jumped back! I had the best chuckle! Who looks like a bull with his balls cut off now!

Working with these kids was draining! We popped into the ICU where my wife had been. The staff was delighted to see me and were equally delighted when they heard how well she was doing. We were transferring their patient who was on a ventilator, and of course I wanted to do my best in front of these guys. I adjusted my ventilator, checked the settings, and we switched the patient over. While I was getting the rest of the report, I could see that the patient's O2 saturation was dropping! I began to reassess, thinking D.O.P.E.: dislodged tube—no, obstruction—no, pneumothorax—no, equipment—yes! My EMT never turned the oxygen supply on. He had one job and failed! I was very happy I was paying attention.

Another call brought me into an ER where the patient was shot in the face. I could see that the nurse had handed him a Yankauer suction device, so he could continually suction his mouth, which was constantly filling up with blood. What I thought a bit interesting was that she was pushing doses of IV fentanyl at the same time. Narcotic sedation with no airway protection could prove to be dangerous! Of course, the fentanyl would eventually decrease his consciousness and respiratory rate and depth, wouldn't it?

I looked at the patient and searched out the doctor. Once I found her, I asked if she was concerned about the patient's neck because the force of the gunshot or possible projectile could have injured his spinal cord. Together we looked at his x-ray, which revealed the shattered bone and the bullet. However, it appeared his neck was clear. I then inquired about his airway status. I said, "You know, we do have a potential airway problem." I told the doctor I could manage his airway en route, though it might require me to stop and intubate. I said, "You know, they are going to intubate him at the trauma center."

She then looked at me and said, "Sometimes it's good to have a fresh set of eyes looking in on a case." With that, I set up our ventilator. We pushed the paralytics, hung some Propofol, and the patient was tubed and transported.

CHAPTER 38

THE PAIN OF LOSS

Our patient was a seven-year-old girl with cerebral palsy. We were called to transfer her to a university hospital that had a pediatric ICU bed available for her. Before arriving, I had received a report that indicated that the patient was in a considerable amount of respiratory distress. I was concerned about the potential of respiratory failure. I was wondering why the girl wasn't intubated and ventilated. When I arrived, my suspicions proved true. The girl's mother was calling all the shots. There was no way she wanted her daughter on the ventilator. Her rationale was that the last time her baby was on a ventilator, it was too difficult to get her off! Everything inside me wanted to tell her that respiratory failure leads to cardiovascular collapse and death, but I kept my mouth shut.

I looked at the patient's blood gas, which revealed a CO_2 of 200. I've never seen a number like that before. The normal range is between 35 and 45. I spoke to the ER doctor, but there was no way that they wanted to push the issue. Truth be told, the intubation would not be an easy one. I stepped back to assess my options. I was seriously considering declining the transport.

I knew how it was going to go. I would be on the road for two hours working in a frenzy to keep the patient alive, thinking there would be an excellent chance she would arrive at the receiving hospital dead. I really did not want that experience.

The nurse was giving me report and additional background information. As she was talking, I was reading her nursing notes and noticed her last name on the bottom of the chart. It was Lucy! I had no clue! We had worked and flown together for years. We sat next to each other on hundreds of flights and yet I didn't recognize her right in front of me! We had the best laugh. I guess we'd both changed after all those years! We got a bit older! I looked back at the patient and her mother. I knew that getting her to the university hospital was their only chance. So, against my better judgement, I said "Fuck it." We loaded the patient in the ambulance and had her mom sitting up front. I didn't want her in the back getting in my way. The transfer was just as I had expected. I spent the whole two hours suctioning her airway. At the same time, I had the EMT watching the pulse oximeter to alert me when the O2 saturation dropped below 90. At that point, I would ventilate the patient's O2 saturation back up. Once the saturation was in the 90s, I would suction her again. I went through every suction catheter we had on the rig. It was a constant back and forth between suction, ventilation, suction, ventilation. I was sweating buckets. The EMT was freaking out. He had never seen anyone work so intently. There was no way this patient was going to die on my transfer!

We got to the pediatrics ICU and the staff's eyes were bulging in disbelief. The resident looked at me, and I shook my head as I gave her the patient's last blood gas. The resident then tried to assess lung sounds and I told her there were none! As we transferred the patient to her bed, the resident was trying to explain to the mother that they needed to intubate immediately.

The mother said no. Sometimes, the reality of having to let go is just too painful, too heartbreaking. We gathered our equipment, I washed my hands and face, and we left.

I recalled an older Asian man. He and his wife were driving when their car was T-boned. The man's wife was killed, and he was discharged from the ER without a scratch. He asked me, "What am I going to do now? She did everything for me." I had no answer for him. We hugged, and I led him to the door. I still remember his face, I remember his tears.

On the way back to quarters, I also recalled my own father's funeral. I remember the undertaker wheeling him out of the house in a purple body bag. When we were leaving his gravesite, I heard my mother cry. It was no ordinary cry. It was deep and cutting. I knew it was bad and that my childhood was over. I remember crying like that when my grandfather passed away.

A young man was in a verbal altercation, beaten, and ended up in the ICU with a traumatic brain injury. He was on life support. His wife was broken, and the family was in insurmountable grief. We transferred him to another hospital for organ donation. The wife asked the physician to harvest the man's viable sperm. She wanted a baby, and the family did not want to lose their boy. The facility complied.

We rolled up to a nursing home where we were to take a patient to the ER. I found the man's daughter there in tears. She told me that her father had been fine yesterday. He was awake, alert, and talking. They had a great visit. Now the man was unresponsive. He had a fever and was hypoxic. We began to load him up and get him on oxygen when she asked me if I would transfer him to the hospital with the sirens on. I told her I would treat her father like he was my father. As she cried, we hugged. We ran Code 3! Grief, it's the price of love. It's not cheap.

CHAPTER 39

BREAKING POINTS

Starting another 24-hour shift on the ambulance, I was receiving report from the departing crew. I had one foot up on the step when an EMT reached between my legs and grabbed my genitals. I turned around and yelled, "Don't ever do that again!" All the while, I'm looking at the angle of his jaw, ready to throw my fist at it. A 25-year-old punk just grabbed a 60-year-old man's junk! Who does that? I walked into the administrative office to file the complaint, but nothing ever came of it. These kids were empowered to behave as they pleased. I remembered I had been fired once for not fighting, and I really didn't want to lose another job.

We were called for a transfer to the city. The patient was in end-stage liver failure. She was sick, on a ventilator and on vasopressors, most likely not going to survive the trip. Still, the city hospital was her only hope! It was a Friday and we were moving into rush hour traffic. I calculated our oxygen supply against what the patient would need. The only way we could make it was if we ran Code 3, lights and sirens all the way into the city. We took off.

We flew into the ambulance entrance of the receiving hospital and transferred the patient to the ICU. There, I was met by the senior resident. The look on his face was priceless. He said, "We heard your siren."

I said, "Yeah, we're coming in hot!" He was thinking I was either crazy or had some big balls to transport this woman. Honestly, it was a little bit of both.

We stopped to grab some lunch. The EMT I was with always had a habit of slugging or pushing me. On this particular day, I had enough, and I asked him to stop. I said, "You know, one day you're going to hit me and I'm going to hit you back." Now, I'm not sure if he thought I was joking or if he wanted to find out. As I turned away, he pushed me again. Well, I turned and threw a ridge hand strike right at his Adam's apple. I struck him perfectly, with just enough force to get his larynx to spasm a bit. I needed to make a point. A ridge hand strike is an old karate hand offensive strike. It was frequently used in tournaments back in the 70s. It stopped him in his tracks and he began coughing. For a while, he couldn't move. After that, he never touched me. Don't mess with an old man.

Another EMT ran around the quarters with 30 cc syringes filled with water. He'd pull the syringe from his pants through the zipper and act as if he were masturbating. He then would shoot the saline all over the staff, equipment, and furniture. Somehow, I was to find this funny. I was working with idiots.

One shift, I was running calls all day and night. I had cardiac patients, stroke patients, ventilated patients, and one right after the other. It was nonstop. Finally, we were on our way back to the quarters with 15 minutes left of our shift. We were off at 8 AM. The pager sounded, and we were routed out of the county. It would be a long transfer. Our 24-hour shift had just been extended to 34 hours. I was toast. We turned the rig around, filled up with gas, and proceeded to the sending facility. After about 10 minutes in transit, the EMT in the back started laughing his ass off. Turned out he was the one sending the page as a joke. It was then that I was convinced my time trying to work with these kids had to come to an end.

Luckily, I had some old friends who had informed me that there was an open spot in their ICU. I was thinking that perhaps now would be the time to make the change. Without hesitation, I called the manager. We had a great interview and he was happy to hire, as he put it, a "seasoned nurse."

CHAPTER 40

OVERCOOKED

It was my last day, and what a day it was. The first call was an obstetrics run. High-risk labor and preterm labor always elevated my awareness and anxiety. I knew I needed a lot of luck and had to be ready for anything.

On a flight years ago, the mother was in preterm labor and had a condition called polyhydramnios. She was filled with an abnormal amount of amniotic fluid. The baby was at risk, and we had to get her to the city. The flight went well, but the ambulance ride to the hospital was a bit sketchy. At one point, she said she needed to go to the bathroom. I slid her a bedpan. I was beginning to freak out, I had to look under her gown. I was just praying there was no bulging, no crowning, and please no baby!

A few moments later, her membranes broke. Now, I'm not talking about a bag of water. It was as if someone had poured out two five-gallon bottles of Arrowhead drinking water. As the ambulance coursed through the streets, waves of amniotic fluid were sloshing all around us. My flight suit was soaked! I never saw so much fluid.

We got the patient up to the ninth floor and into her bed. Back at the rig, I couldn't find my pager, so I called the upstairs unit to see if I left it on their counter. The nurse said she couldn't look for it right now because they were delivering the woman's baby! Man, I had an angel on my shoulder!

As I walked down the hall to pick up our patient in labor, I ran into Mary. She was a nursing supervisor I knew from one of the hospitals where I'd previously been employed. I liked her a lot. One day, she approached me in that ER and said she wanted to ask me a question. She said, "You know you're different than the staff down here. You're always smiling, always happy while your co-workers here are always so negative. Why is that?" I looked at her and chuckled. All I could say was, "If you see any good in me, it's God's work through me. It ain't me!"

Mary replied, "Well, it shows." I thought that was a really nice thing to hear. Then I thought, "Maybe I did get to be a little like that nurse Anna. Maybe I am a bit set apart."

Seeing Mary in the hall was very nice. We gave each other a big hug as she turned to her staff and said, "You see that guy? He's a nurse's nurse!" What a compliment! Maybe one of the best I ever received!

It was another long day. Early the next morning, we picked up a woman in respiratory distress. She was in congestive heart failure and on BiPAP. She wanted to get off the breathing machine, so I told her we could try. I took her off the BiPAP and moved her to the gurney. She instantly became shorter of breath, so back on the mask and machine she went.

The receiving hospital was only about 15 minutes away. As we were leaving, the sending nurse called to give them report. Once we were en route, we called the receiving ER as well and gave them our ETA. Upon arrival, the receiving nurse was perched on her chair and never looked up from her phone. Then she asked, "Did we know she was coming?" I was wiped out and not really in the best mood. There was no introduction, and she didn't even look at the patient. I knew they were called twice.

We finally got the patient into a room. The nurse walked straight to her computer with her back to us and eventually said, "Okay, you can give me report now." Over the course of the information exchange, she would interrupt repeatedly. At one point, she had asked me if I tried to get the lady off BiPAP. It was an odd question because we ordinarily don't mess with much during transport. Ironically, though, we did try to take her off the BiPAP this time. I told the nurse as much and she responded, "Well, how did she do?" I looked at the patient, then back at the nurse whose back was still to us and said, "Well, she's still on it!" One of her colleagues looked at me and called me an asshole. I wanted to have a private chat with him.

We were 23 hours into our shift with one hour to go. We got a call that took us deep into the city, to a care home with ventilated patients. I had all the equipment set up. We entered the home just moments after their shift change, and no one could give me a detailed report. No one, I mean no one, knew anything about the patient. All I could gather was that he was a traumatic brain injured patient. He was trached on a ventilator with a fever and high blood sugar. He'd also been given some insulin. We loaded him up and transported.

At the receiving ER, the triage nurse was saying, "We know nothing about this patient." I showed her the paperwork with the accepting MD and gave her report. With that, she started making phone calls and running around the department. I had the patient tied up in a gurney and our O2 was burning. I asked for a bed, but she ignored me. I turned to my crew and began, "Do you see this? This is an excellent example of patient-centered care. This nurse will keep us waiting and keep the patient all tied up. It doesn't matter, they are going to accept the patient. They have to." We stood there for one hour and then I gave report to another triage nurse.

Finally, we got to a room. A nurse showed up and I gave him report. As I was talking, he kept interrupting me. He had a group of staff behind him. The report went as follows: "The patient is a 25-year-old male with a head injury. He is a five on the Glasgow Coma Scale and his temperature is 102°F." They gave Tylenol.

The nurse asked, "What's his temperature?"

I replied, "102°F." I then told the nurse that the patient's blood sugar was 270 and they administered six units of insulin. He then asked why they checked his blood sugar and I replied, "I don't know." He inquired about the patient's blood sugar and I said, "270." He then repeated his question about the insulin, so I said, "Man, I just told you six units!"

Someone in the back yells, "Hey, you don't have to get all aggressive!" I looked back at him, looked at the nurse, and knew I had to get out of there. Finally, one of the bystanders walked in and helped us transport the patient to the bed.

I was in that ER for 90 minutes, gave report three times, and somehow, I was the bad guy. We got out of there and not a moment too soon. The shift was over, and I was going home, but not before coffee. I really needed a good cup of coffee. We stopped at a coffee shop and I got the biggest latte they served. On the road home, I took a sip of the warm latte that I'd been dreaming of, only to get a mouthful of coffee with soured milk! Well, fuck me!

I gave my notice and was wrapping up one of my last shifts. We got a call about a pretty sick patient, and I recognized the name. It was a nurse I used to work with. I really liked her. She was sick and most likely going to die. I wasn't looking forward to the call. I got there, saw her, and said I would do whatever she needed to keep her comfortable. I was surprised to see that her nurse was one I knew also. It was nurse video game. I guess she got a new job. As I was beginning to load the patient, she came up behind me and pressed herself against me. I was thinking, "You've got to be kidding me, as crazy as you are?" I couldn't get out of there fast enough. The transfer was smooth, and I did all I could for her. En route, she asked me how my wife was doing. I was blown away that even with her pain and end-stage disease she showed concern for my wife and me.

CHAPTER 41

BACK IN THE SADDLE

So, I jumped back into the ICU. It was going to be easy money. There were three 12-hour shifts a week, and I could sleep again. It was all good.

I'm working with a guy who seemed nice enough. As I arrived, he was bumped up into a management position. He began to orient me when he stepped out of the unit and never came back! After that, it was obvious that I was on my own. I took my time fumbling through their electronic health record and figured it out.

The shifts were easy. I enjoyed the work, and it didn't take too long to figure out that the new manager was worthless. He spent the majority of his time on the computer watching his old surf break, Bell's Beach! One day, we were working the unit together. I was caring for my patient as he got an admission. Now, I knew the patient and the family he was admitting. John made no effort to go over there, so I approached the family and did the admission. They were all quite concerned about their grandmother.

They expressed their concerns about the care their grandmother was not receiving at the nursing home. They pointed out that she had developed a bed sore. I assessed it, grabbed some dressings for it, and gave my report to John along with the dressing. I had to get back to my patient. Two hours later, the admitting physician came in and talked to the family. He then approached John and said that the family would really like the dressing over her bed sore! I was blown away! Who is this guy? He ignored the patient and the family for hours!

I walked in one day to find him training a new nurse. She was fresh out of school and very cute. It was no wonder he stayed beside her.

An older female patient was post-op, out of bed, and off the cardiac monitor. John left the young nurse alone to care for her. About the same time, the patient's daughter approached me and said, "My mom does not feel well." I walked over to find her cold and pale. We lifted her up onto the bed and I placed her back on the cardiac monitor to find her in a supraventricular tachycardia (a very rapid heart rate in the 160s). Her blood pressure was fine, so I opened the crash cart and pushed some adenosine, a medication that would break the rapid rate. The intensive care doctor walked in and whispers in my ear, "Thank you." The sad part was that John left the young nurse to flounder. She felt so inadequate, she quit.

As time went on, I was pushed into co-managing with John. I didn't want anything to do with it, but they were forcing their hand. John was going on a two-week vacation and brought me up to speed on where he was at with things. He asked me to make some fliers, since he was scheduling a staff meeting upon his return.

While he was gone, I hit the ground running. I was watching over the ICU and the emergency room, putting little fires out everywhere. It was fine. I got a call from John, inquiring about the staff meeting agenda! "What agenda?" I asked. He was the one who called the meeting. I had just distributed the fliers as he'd directed me to. I told him there were a few things I needed to talk about and that I had put together a PowerPoint presentation at the request of the admitting department. He asked to see the presentation, so I e-mailed it him. John made some revisions on my presentation and asked me which part of it I wanted to do. I was a bit taken aback. What part of my presentation did I want to do? I told him I really didn't care.

Upon his return from vacation, we had the staff meeting. It was a joke! Halfway through the agenda, while I was speaking, John stepped up and took over. I never got to finish what I was saying. He then introduced his wife, who worked there as an educator. She began to deliver my PowerPoint presentation! I was blown away! I looked over at the director of nursing and told her, "I'm not working with this guy."

She looked straight at me and said, "Fuck you!"

Since the ICU position I had was filled, I jumped back into a float position. I was asked to do some training for the new nurses that they hired in the emergency department. I was happy to do it!

We scheduled a time to go over the topic of emergency cardiac care. I began with the basics of emergency care and then delved into stable and unstable cardiac arrhythmias. We discussed the current treatments, etc. I always found this life-saving information quite fascinating. As I scanned the audience, much of the staff were focused on their cell phones. I just didn't get it. Trying to educate this group, who ironically thought they were "the shit," proved to be for me an impossibility to teach let alone inspire. How unfortunate.

I walked into the ER one day to find a few patients waiting. Among them was a woman with some psychiatric issues who was being ignored. Another patient was complaining about heart palpitations. I took the patient with psychiatric issues. We had a good conversation. As I triaged her, I assured her she would get the help she needed, and things would get better for her. I then arrived back in the main room to hear alarms beeping. The nurse who triaged the patient with palpitations was sitting next to me gabbing away. I told her, "You know your patient's heart rate is pretty fast."

She responded, "It's not that fast; it's only 160." I got up to have a look at the patient. There was no IV and no EKG. I placed the IV line, drew her blood, then asked the ER technician to do the EKG and grab the doctor. We pushed Cardizem and started a drip to slow the patient's heart rate down. I got the patient admitted to the ICU. I couldn't really look at that ER nurse. I felt she was worthless.

I recalled another time when I received report from her. She told me that her patient was getting some IV potassium and going home. I went to see the patient to find the potassium was not on an IV pump, and the patient was not on a cardiac monitor! I told the patient I was going to place the potassium on a pump and, if she didn't mind, I'd hook her up to the cardiac monitor. She was fine with it. Well, I found her in a supraventricular tachycardia (SVT) at 180 beats per minute. I told the doctor that the patient was in SVT and she asked, "You know this how?" I told her I saw it on the monitor! We slowed her down, cardiology saw her, and she was admitted to the ICU. As I wheeled her to her room, she turned to me and said, "You saved my life."

I laughed a bit and said, "I don't know about that, but your cardiologist is going to take very good care of you!"

Back in the ER, I went out to the triage desk where I found a woman in what looked to be excruciating pain! The look on her face said it all. I asked her why she came in, and it turned out that she'd just been discharged from the hospital. She informed me that she had had a labial cyst that was cut open, drained, and packed. She was miserable and could hardly even walk. I brought her back and got her into a room when the doctor approached me. Now, I've known this particular doctor for years. She was absolutely horrible! She asked me why the patient was there, and I told her. The doctor then began screaming in the middle of the ER, five feet from the patient's bed, "Why is she here? She was just discharged! She had follow-up appointments!"

I looked at her and said, "I didn't tell her to come in!" I walked away from her and reported the incident to the medical director. Of course, nothing ever happened. The patient, I'm sure, felt less than human! Sometimes, I just don't know.

The next triage was a female patient who was cold and clammy. She had a urine analysis that revealed infection. I couldn't find the doctor, so I started an IV, drew all the blood, and sent it to the lab. I was giving report to another nurse, and as I left the doctor approached me. She was screaming that I should have come to her first since she needed to write the orders! All I could think was, "You would have the right to scream at me if I just walked away from a septic patient and didn't do anything. You're yelling at me because I did my job?" I looked her up and down, turned my head back to the nurse, and said "I got both sets of blood cultures, too!" I walked away, reflecting that times sure have changed over the years. The world has just gotten crazier.

CHAPTER 42

IT'S ALWAYS WHO YOU KNOW

As time passed, my wife was becoming weaker and weaker at an earlier point each day. The virus that had attacked her heart weakened and dilated the muscle to a point where it simply didn't pump well. You could compare it to an overstretched rubber band, it just wouldn't snap back. After further evaluation, it was decided that she would need an implanted pacemaker to resynchronize her heartbeat. We travelled to the city and met with a great physician. She was scheduled the procedure in two weeks! Yet somehow, insurance found a way to interfere. Their stance was that they would insure the hospital, but not the doctor! Everyone was in an uproar, me included! I was thinking, if her health was compromised because of insurance games, I wasn't sure what my response would be. Finally, the doctor said, "Screw them, I will put it in free. Just get her down here!"

Insurance said, "No way!" We were stuck!

We were then referred to another physician, but it would be two months before we could see him. He worked at a hospital where an old friend of mine was the ER director. I called Dan, and we had a nice chat. He knew the doctor we were to see. I told him we couldn't wait the two months and asked him to do anything he could. We hung up. An hour later, my phone rang. We had an appointment to see this new doctor the next day. Three days later, my wife had the pacemaker implanted. I was the happiest, most grateful man in the world. It was just like the day when I was a kid and I got to meet Ernie Banks, "Mr. Cub"! He shook my hand and autographed a photo for me. I was the happiest kid in Chicago! Now I was the happiest man in California!

A few weeks later, we were shopping, and I saw Leslie, an ICU nurse with fiery red hair. She was in her car, about to pull away, when I tapped on her window. When she saw me, her eyes bugged out. I pointed to my wife, who she cared for in the hospital. Leslie ran out of the car and gave her the biggest hug. It was awesome. I saw her tears of joy!

As if that wasn't enough, my wife and I went to grab a cup of coffee a few days later. Outside the café was Kathy, the finest nurse I've ever known! What a moment. We sat down, and I didn't say a word. These two people just looked at each other. My wife had no clue what kind of care Kathy had taken of her, but I did. I couldn't wipe the tears off my face fast enough. Kathy said it was the first time she had ever met a patient outside of work. It was the sweetest moment; it was meant to be!

CHAPTER 43

WHAT'S WRONG WITH PEOPLE?

Back in the ER, I'm helping out when we receive a patient who is going through alcohol withdrawal. The only people present were me, the doctor, and another nurse.

I worked the patient up. He was to receive IV fluids, Ativan to quiet the withdrawal symptoms, and an infusion of vitamins. I stepped out to go to the bathroom and returned to find all the IVs disconnected on my patient. I asked the other nurse about it and she ignored me. I asked her again and she put her hand up in my face. Apparently, she decided to discontinue the IV fluids on my patient on her own. I couldn't believe what I was seeing! Who does that?

Another day, I'm assigned to relieve the same nurse for a lunch break. She begins to leave without giving me any report apart from saying that she has a patient who is coming back from x-ray for his hip since he had fallen. She had been caring for him in the department for two hours. The patient returned from x-ray hypoxic, so I gave him oxygen. I then placed him on a cardiac monitor and found him bradycardic with a heart rate of 27 per minute in a third-degree AV block (a malfunction of the cardiac electrical conduction system). I immediately grabbed the doctor. The patient was sent to the catheterization lab for a pacemaker. The nurse returned from lunch, wondering where her patient went. I told her.

A doctor was in the ICU, moving from patient to patient without washing her hands. It was disgusting. One of the patients she saw was on contact precautions due to Clostridium difficile (C. diff). I kindly asked her to wash her hands and observe the precautions when she started going off on me. After all, who was I but a nurse? I stood up to her and informed her that I would always advocate for my patients. I asked her if she understood. We were never very good friends after that!

The following case was especially sad. I really wished I could have done something, anything, sooner. A 45-year-old man entered the ICU escorted by one of the ER nurses. His wife was also nurse. I just needed to look at her face, she got it.

The ER nurse tells us he's fine, his vitals are stable! I could see the patient was only focusing on what was right in front of him. He was breathing at about 60 and the respirations were deep and fast. I checked his radial pulse and it was absent. The ER nurse was not helping! The IV lines were badly tangled. It was a mess. I moved the patient over to the bed as the nurse repeatedly asked me if I knew what she wanted to tell me. She was making no sense. They had the patient for four and a half hours, and it was just now that she was trying to hang his antibiotic. I wanted her out of the unit. She was only getting in the way.

I got the patient hooked up, started a 14 g IV, opened up IV fluids, and set up for a central line. Once I was finished, I called the doctor in stat! We started a vasopressor, Levophed, and began to dial in the patient's blood pressure. He was a diabetic with an overwhelming infection. I labored over this man for hours, to no avail. I watched him die. I wish I had those four and a half hours that were spent in the ER. Maybe, just maybe, that time would have made a difference. That day, a nurse lost her husband and her kids lost their father. There are no do-overs!

Another patient was in the bed next door. He was an older man with bad atherosclerosis. He had had a left lower extremity amputation as a result. He had been admitted because his right foot was not being perfused. It was cold and blue, and the Doppler revealed no pulses. It was possibly time to start cutting again. His vasculature was full of plaque!

I noticed that he had atrial fibrillation and the rate was picking up, so I called his doctor. I figured he'd need some IV medication to control his heart rate. As I step into the room and pulled the curtain back, I found another nurse giving him a bilateral carotid sinus massage! She was literally mashing down on the two plaque-filled arteries that ordinarily feed his brain with oxygen-rich blood! The man was lucky to have survived her without a big stroke! I was looking around wondering, "What the hell is wrong with people?"

I worked with another nurse who was a typical control freak ICU nurse. She was overseeing the care of a man who was a bit demented and would get combative at times. She wouldn't leave him alone. The patient was fine lying in bed, but Jackie was intent on getting him up. I had offered to help, but as usual she replied that she had it! In no time at all, push came to shove. She wanted him up, and he wanted to get back to bed. As they began to wrestle, he shat all over the floor. Jackie was in a state of panic. Both she and the patient were stepping in the shit and it was getting all over the place! I came over and got the guy back in bed. By this time, he was so worked up that we were going to have to restrain him. Jackie approached him without thinking and caught a side kick to the ribs. She went flying across the room into a table, but never went down. I was thinking, "Damn! She could take a shot!" She took a couple weeks off after that happened.

I was walking back into the ER one day and overheard a nurse yelling at a patient. Apparently, he had a habit of dislocating his shoulder and needed surgery. He never scheduled an appointment with the orthopedic surgeon. Instead, he'd just come back to the ER to get it fixed. The nurse was tired of him and screamed, "If you do this again, we will not take care of you!" Now, I have no idea what any of the other patients thought of the outburst, but I imagine it wasn't a good reflection of the ER, the hospital, or nursing for that matter.

I was beginning to think that the place was way too out of control. The staff was clueless and some of the doctors seemed way out there also. I spent some time reflecting on my experience in some of the other hospitals and on the ambulances. The whole situation seemed hopeless. I wasn't sure that there was any place left for me to turn. I was beginning to feel stuck; I was running out of options.

Since Jackie was out, I worked in the ICU more often and that was good for me. I could take care of my patients and do what I felt was a good job. After a few weeks, Jackie returned. She was scheduled to work the ICU with an orientee, and I was scheduled to be the house supervisor. She called me at home the night before and asked if I would switch with her. She said she would do house supervisor if I would orient the new nurse. Her rationale was that she was out so long, she wouldn't know what to do. She was out two weeks, but I agreed. That morning, Jackie spent most of her time with me in the ICU. She said she knew nothing about house supervision and proceeded to spend the next four hours complaining about the hospital. Sometime around 11 AM, she looked at me and asked if I was okay. I told her that I was okay, but after listening to her complain all morning, I wasn't doing too well!

Finally, they figured that the ICU manager was useless, and he was fired. His wife, the hospital educator, immediately walked out of a class she was teaching once she got the news that her husband was let go. Two days later, the director of nursing quit. The hospital was rudderless. The ICU admissions would slow down, and I would be called off frequently to spend time at home on call at a third of my hourly wage. Things were not looking promising. I was there for a year, and the landscape looked bleak. I really wanted to settle in and do a few more years, finishing my nursing career on a positive note. I wasn't sure how I was going to make it to the finish line. I spoke to the intensivist, who desperately wanted me to stay, but I explained to him that it was a monetary issue and that I had to look elsewhere.

The truth is that I raised a family on a nurse's salary all these years. Had I stayed back at the old county place, I'd be in a better position to retire. Moving around and bouncing from place to place over the years wasn't the way to build a solid retirement. I still had to work, I still had to earn. Maybe it was true: nursing would chew me up and spit me out when there was nothing left of me.

CHAPTER 44

TRY IT AGAIN

It was back to the job search, looking online and filling out the applications. I have to admit, it was a bit exhausting and I was beginning to feel that I was looking for something that just wasn't there; it just did not exist. All I really wanted was to find an ER where I could do my job to the best of my abilities and work in relative peace. I was dreaming.

I received a call from an ER manager. He sounded perfect over the phone. His voice carried energy and rang out positivity. It was refreshing. I had an appointment to meet with him, and I was very optimistic. The sound of his voice convinced me that I could work for him. We met, and in no time at all he said, "I want to offer you the position." I was delighted!

The hiring process was smooth. I was keeping my fingers crossed that my previous firing wouldn't come back to haunt me. Fortunately, it didn't. I did, however, get a call from HR with a question about my application. They needed clarification about my graduation date from nursing school. Apparently, I listed the month as May when it was January. I told her I couldn't remember the month, it was 32 years ago after all!

I was scheduled for orientation, so I prepared myself to spend the day on the computer. After a few hours, I was told I could finish the shift in the ER. I had no way of knowing I'd be working until 7 PM that evening. I was never informed. They gave me some scrubs, I grabbed some lunch, and began my day.

Now, what I've found over the years is that ER nursing actually becomes easier. Maybe that's the way it is with all jobs—the longer you do them, the more experience you gain. The skills you acquire all make the work easier.

I received a patient who met what are called the systematic inflammatory response syndrome (SIRS) criteria. His vital signs were a bit out of whack, he had a fever, and his heart rate was up. He also had a cough, which seemed to indicate the presence of an infection. The doctor saw him and ordered the usual labs and IV fluids. As I was gathering supplies, I grabbed an IV pole. A nurse named Mike (he'd been there for 30 years) stopped me in my tracks and asked me why I was grabbing an IV pole. I told him I was hanging fluids, to which he responded, "You know there's a pole on the gurney."

What I wanted to say was, "Really? I've been pushing gurneys for 35 years. You think I would have noticed." Clearly, he wanted to establish his territory. I couldn't go through it again, so I told him, "This pole goes higher, that way the fluid can run in faster." I asked him where the pressure cables were for the monitor. My patient had a central line and I wanted to measure his central venous pressure (CVP).

His response was, "Cables?" He laughed and walked away. Again, I could tell something was off with this guy, something was wrong. In no time at all, I got the impression that he was a bully and had no problem trying to push me around. It was also clear that he didn't care at all about patients. I was wondering how in the hell he kept his job or why he was even a nurse in the first place.

I remember he received a patient who was altered. I went into the room to help him get the workup done. I did the IV and drew the patient's blood. Then the patient was taken to do a CT scan. Mike let him go unattended, which was an unsafe action, so I ran to CT to keep an eye on the patient. Five minutes later, he shows up saying, "I'll watch him, you need to go back to the ER. There's a patient in triage." I had to laugh. This guy would do anything to get out of working any harder.

As we neared the end of the shift, things were beginning to wind down. As always, we wanted to get out on time. It was just about 10 minutes before the end of the shift and two patients presented in triage. I saw Mike scurry down the hallway to the front desk. He came walking back with a patient who looked like he had no business coming to the ER. As they approached, Mike told me there was an eye emergency out there waiting! I was a bit stupefied! Working in an ER, it's always life and limb! He was willing to delay the care of a patient with an eye emergency just so he could get home on time! Who does that?

I had been in the ER a very short time and I already began to feel that I'd made a big mistake. Nothing felt right, and it was apparent I would need a coat of armor if I was going to stay and try to make this place my home.

CHAPTER 45

ARE YOU KIDDING ME?

I remember a manager I worked with once told me that I cared too much. One of the nurses I worked with was upset with me and said I treated everyone like an emergency. I could never understand these remarks. I worked in a caring profession and did my time in an emergency room. Wasn't I supposed to care and work intently? Maybe they were right, though. It's possible I would have been better off being more apathetic regarding patients and their care. Certainly, my adrenaline surges didn't do much to help my blood pressure. But honestly, I liked being an ER nurse. It somehow suited me, and I relished the challenges of the emergencies. I always felt like I was in my element. The busier it got, the more out of control it got, the more I liked it. Perhaps my problem was that I could never stay in my lane, I don't know.

Another shift with Mike revealed that he really didn't care much for the homeless, addicts, or alcoholics. It seemed like the guy hated everybody, including the staff and the hospital! He had a young female patient who was going through alcohol withdrawal. She was shaking and unsteady on her feet. I saw her walking to the bathroom and I was a bit concerned. I looked at Mike and said, "Man, she needs more Ativan."

He told me that she'd received one milligram. Clearly, it wasn't touching her, so I asked him if we had a withdrawal protocol and suggested we reference it and alert the physician. Mike's response was, "Ah, she's a drinker." There wasn't too much I could do because I was loaded up with patients. All I did was observe Mike sitting at the nurse's station ignoring his patient. The girl spent seven hours in the ER because the unit wouldn't be staffed until the night shift. By the time the girl got to the ICU, she ended up completely sedated and placed on a ventilator. Under Mike's care, she fell into full-blown delirium tremens (DTs).

I couldn't let it go. I care too much. I placed a call to my manager and tried to get some direction. I asked him what I should do if I noticed patients were not getting the care they deserved. He told me to come to him and he would take care of it. I thought, "Fair enough." He began to press me about what prompted my question. I really did not want to get into it. I did recite my observation about the young girl in withdrawal, but he wanted names. I was reluctant to go further and told him I was only looking for direction. He then demanded names. Seeing as he was my boss, I gave up the goods. Man, did I get an earful. He went off about how he wanted Mike gone. He complained that HR was no help. I was hearing things I wasn't meant to hear, but I came away with the clear sense that he wanted him gone!

Apparently, Mike was called in to HR and confronted about the incident. Unfortunately, I somehow managed to get drawn into it. Afterwards, the manager said Mike's story was different from mine. I just looked at him. All he needed to do was look at the patient and the chart.

Needless to say, there was a bit of love lost between Mike and me. I really didn't care, but I knew that he had a few friends in the ER and his wife held an administrative role. Things could get tricky for me.

Nursing students would come through the ER. Without exception, they were assigned to me. I had a ball with these students. I would teach them everything I could: airway

management, emergency cardiac care, pediatric assessment, everything. One day, I was going through the defibrillator with a student and a nurse named Pam joined us. Pam was an interesting lady. She was lazy and would never stop eating. She also had one heck of an attitude. Pam was Mike's friend.

As I was talking to the student, Pam began to butt in and interrupt. I was handling it without issue. At one point, she asked me how long I depressed the button on the machine during a synchronized cardioversion. I replied, "Hell, I don't know. I hit the button, and it shocks on the R wave." Anyway, I got back to the student.

Mary was one of the nursing instructors. I knew her from way back. She had come into the department and copied my schedule to make sure her students were assigned to me whenever I was working. I enjoyed the students quite a bit. The manager was also assigning new nurses to me to precept. Mike and Pam, who had been there for years, obviously weren't too fond of that fact.

My 90-day evaluation was upon me. The manager called me in to review it. Everything was fine. Then he told me that I needed to work on my technical skills. I was told I was misinforming students.

He said I should be referencing educational material and ensuring that the material I was teaching was accurate. I had no idea what he was talking about! I pressed him to be specific, so he referenced a conversation he had with Pam in which Pam stated I didn't know how to operate a defibrillator!

I looked at him straight in the eye and asked, "Are you kidding me?" I inquired if I was being counseled on how long to depress a button on the defibrillator? I told him I didn't even know how to respond.

He caught my eye and, in that instant, seemed to recognize he was being played. He shook his head and said, "You know, I should have come to you first and talked to you." I will delete this off your evaluation. I shook my head. I'd been an ER nurse for over 30 years and taught ACLS for the better part of 25 years only to be faced with this!

Two days later, there was a cardiac arrest on the floor. I ran down there to find CPR in progress. The patient had tracheostomy, so the airway was good. She had one small IV line. I placed the patient on the monitor and saw ventricular fibrillation on the screen. I charged the defibrillator, yelled "clear!", and shocked the patient. I suggested epinephrine. The doctor arrived and was calling out orders. I gave the epinephrine. We shocked again, dosed the patient with amiodarone, continued the CPR, and shocked again. The patient went into Torsades de pointes, so I pulled up the magnesium and administered it. I set up the central line for the doctor as he placed a right internal jugular line. We gave more epinephrine, shocked, and had a tachycardia with pulses. I checked the blood pressure with a Doppler. The patient's blood pressure was in the 60s. Fluids were opened up, and I suggested Levophed.

We stabilized the patient. She was moved to the ER, where I managed her on a Levophed and an amiodarone drip. We replaced her potassium and magnesium. I was keeping an eye on her CVP (I found the pressure cables that Mike laughed about).

I was watching her mean arterial pressure (MAP) and dialing her vital signs in perfectly. The patient's mother was right beside me now. My manager walked in, looked at me, and said, "You are a real asset to this hospital."

I wanted to say, "It's a good thing I know how to work a defibrillator!" Instead, I said "Thank you." I love ER nursing!

I was back in the ER with Mike. He gets a sick-looking older man. The patient had multiple surgeries and was a mess. I was looking at the monitor and could see the pulse oximeter wave was funky. It reminded me of a patient I covered way back whose heart rate was half that on the screen. I mentioned the oddity to Mike, but he paid no mind. The ER tech was telling Mike that the doctor had ordered the patient to be placed on the cardiac monitor, but Mike would not make any effort. In fact, he said that he did put the patient on the monitor and that he had run a cardiac rhythm strip! Now, this made no sense. Who would put a patient on a monitor, run a strip, then take him off? The truth is that Mike never did such a thing. He was lying his ass off!

Finally, I hooked up the patient to the monitor. I found the man to be in what they call ventricular bigeminy. His ventricle was firing as a pacemaker every other beat! Now Mike was trying to convince me it was atrial! I said to him, "Are you telling me that these wide bizarre waves are atrial?" There was no end with this guy! Atrial beats are narrow. Anyone who has taken an EKG class knows that's the case!

I ran a strip and gave it to the ER doctor. Now she was so full of herself, she had to enter the ER through the double doors to fit! I immediately got the impression there was never any reason for her to hear anything I ever had to say. She looked at the arrhythmia and said, "I'm not going to do anything about that." I was thinking, "You've got to be kidding me! Here we go again!"

I shook my head, thinking "Man, these people!" But like a good little nurse, I just went back and sat on my chair! Damn it! There was no place like that old county hospital! I made a big mistake by leaving there.

Later, I had a man present septic. He was overwhelmed with infection. I began to draw his blood when the doctor came up to me upset, saying she did not order anything. I looked at her, removed my gloves, and walked away. After she saw the patient orders were written, the doctor came up to me and said "I just wanted to see you put your gloves back on again."

CHAPTER 46

HARASSMENT OR WORSE

It's always been my tendency to work with a bit of mania, if you will. I guess that's why the pace of the ER appealed to me. When I was a kid, I worked in a factory. I cut tin for all kinds of cans, from coffee cans to tuna cans. It was mindless, and it was fun. The guys I worked with were getting mad at me because I was bundling about 10 loads a night. I was always trying to beat my previous records. I guess I was making them look bad. One day, the boss came up to me and said, "Your balls must be hanging to the floor!" I had a good laugh. He then told me that production was six loads a night. He wanted me to cut back to six. Since he was the boss, he got six loads. Even earlier, when I was a kid I used to wash dishes at a restaurant and I had a ball. I loved whipping through the bus trays. The owner came back to me one day and accused me of being on drugs. He said that he had never seen anyone work that fast! Somehow, my pace had always been an issue, but not with me.

I was called into the director of nurse's office. I guess Pam had a complaint about me. The director looked at me and said, "Now, I don't know what's going on with you two. Pam came to me, complaining that you're taking too many patients!" I had nothing to say. She then said, "I don't care how long it takes. Just sit there and let her take a patient." The director told me she told Pam it could be worse. I could just sit there and take no patients! You can't write this stuff!

So, I let Pam take a patient and then I took one myself. There was another call for a STAT triage. Normally, I would run out front, but it was Pam's turn! She went out there and began to yell for help. The patient was down and unresponsive. I went out there, helped her lift him on a gurney, and brought him into the department. I hooked him up to the cardiac monitor and started an IV. As I turned and looked, I realized Pam was gone! She went back to the nurse's station and was beginning to feed her face! I told her I was happy to help, but she needed to get back in the room and manage her patient. It didn't go over very well, but she was the one who'd complained!

I was drawing blood with a couple extra sets of blood cultures because the patient was febrile. Pam came up and said, "I'll get all your sharps." I thought that was nice, but odd. When I was done, I went to grab the wrappers and toss them in the garbage, but a little voice in my head told me to look and make sure there were no more needles in my pile of trash. As I picked through the waste, sure enough there was a bloody 18-gauge needle that would have pierced my hand. I did not want to believe that there would have been the slightest chance that Pam left it there intentionally. She would never do such a thing, or would she?

Now, the flow in the ER was always dynamic. It was common to get involved with a really sick patient or you might just see three runny noses. I was informed that Pam was making copies of the census. She wanted to document who was taking more patients, who was working harder. Whatever. The ER technician was informing me that it was Pam's intention to build some kind of case against me. Well, I'd had enough and made my own trek to the HR department. I described my working conditions with Pam's history of going to administration about me, telling the manager I did not know how to operate a defibrillator. Now, she was logging patient census. I was expressing how ridiculous it was to have to work under those conditions. The HR representative said that people tend to use the term "harassment" incorrectly. However, in this case, when someone is intentionally trying to get someone fired, the application of the term is correct. He informed me that he would be speaking to Pam and that if her actions didn't cease, they would most certainly backfire on her.

Now, they say to err is human, but to forgive is divine. I am not one to really hold on to things. As much as I like to forgive and forget, sometimes it's just stupid to do so. I made a mistake, a medication error. The doctor ordered some Compazine for a patient and I thought I read promethazine, which is a medication for treating nausea. I gave the wrong drug and was about to record the incident when Pam said, "Just have the doctor change the order." I thought about it and spoke with the doctor. It was basically the same class of medication, often prescribed for similar symptoms. There really was no harm and no foul to the patient. He changed the order and I went on with my day. The manager approached me the next day to counsel me for making a medication error and failing to write it up! After Pam suggested I speak to the doctor, she went straight to the boss. Fool me once! I felt, as they say, like a sheep among wolves.

It was a Sunday morning, and a woman came in frantic. She'd not had a bowel movement for days and was clearly miserable. I tried my best to assure her that we would be able to take care of her. Pam was attempting to forbid me from performing a soap suds enema. She was adamant that we did not do enemas in the

ER! I just looked at her and asked her to show me the policy. Pam was fuller of shit than the patient.

I asked the patient to assume the position and I placed the hose, raising the bag of warm, soapy water. I was able to get her to pass her stool. After a liter and a half of soapy warm water flowing up into her bowel, she got onto the commode and shat all over the place. Her smile returned, and she skipped out of the ER like the happiest kid in the world. That's what I do! I'm a nurse!

I recalled one other occasion when I gave a patient soap suds enema. She was about 90 years old and sharp as a tack! She was all bound up due to the Vicodin she was taking. Her discs were degenerating, causing her all kinds of back pain. The medication brought her relief, but at the cost of constipation. I got her in position, explained the procedure, and began to advance the tube. The patient began to moan, as it caused her a degree discomfort. I responded, "You'll be okay. You can do this."

The patient turned her head towards me, looked me straight in the eye, and said, "I bet you say that to all the girls." I was speechless! She got me!

About a month later, Pam gave her notice. She was heading back to North Dakota. I am sorry to say that I was really happy to see her go.

I remember a patient I had who needed a urinary catheter. I was about to insert the tube into his penis when he asked if it would hurt. I replied it would be uncomfortable during insertion. While it would be indwelling, he might feel a continued urge to urinate due to the pressure of the inflated balloon on his bladder. After I placed the catheter, he told me it wasn't that bad. He said it actually felt like a second orgasm. He asked me if I ever had two. I didn't feel I needed to respond.

CHAPTER 47

SCREAMING ALARMS

Patients in the ER are often connected to cardiac monitors. These monitors are configured with alarm limits. If any vital signs fall out of their normal range of values, the machines ring. It's a great built-in safety mechanism. The alarms are loud and purposefully so. However, there is a well-documented condition that effects the staff called alarm fatigue. Basically, the alarms go off so often that they are turned off and ignored. You may ask yourself, "Who would do such a thing?"

I'm working with Mike, who has a patient with an alarm sounding to indicate that the oxygen saturation is low. I silenced the alarm and informed him of his patient's condition. He responded by saying that the patient was refusing oxygen! The alarm rings again, and again he makes no effort to visit the patient. The saturation is in the low 80s. I got up, introduced myself to the patient, and explained to her that her oxygen level was low. I told her that we needed to supplement her with a nasal cannula. She informed me that the other nurse just told her to take deeper breaths when the monitor alarmed. Who does that?

By the middle of the shift, the ER was full, and the patient load was lopsided—seven to one to be exact. I was running, and I can't say I knew what Mike was doing. He had a patient who was septic and I guess nothing was happening. The doctor came up to me wondering what was up with Mike. He asked if Mike needed a hand. I looked at him and said, "Hey, I have seven patients, he's got one. I think he's giving himself a hand!" We both had a laugh.

With that, I walked into the room to find an older man lying in a wet sheet and he was covered in shit. His daughters were there, looking quite concerned. There was no sign of Mike. I looked at his girls and introduced myself. We cleaned up their father. I started an IV, drew the blood, placed a urinary catheter, then mixed his antibiotics. By this time, Mike appeared and hung the medicine. Later, as I was walking down the hallway, one of the patient's daughters ran out of the room and gave me a huge hug. That was nice.

Mike received a patient who was altered. The patient may have attempted suicide using alcohol and drugs. The same doctor approached me, and he was pissed. Two hours elapsed and there was no urine toxicology screen. I impressed upon Mike that he could not let this kind of thing happen and began to gather the urinary catheter supplies, when he finally took over. Now, it was common knowledge that Mike didn't care for drug addicts, alcoholics, psychiatric patients, and the homeless. Even so, I really couldn't fathom how he would allow them to die under his nursing care. I just shook my head.

By the end of the day, the doctor was in an uproar. He was going off about Mike, and I encouraged him to talk to the manager. Well he did, and then further enquiries were made. A few more doctors were approached, and it finally came down to me. I simply pointed to the patient census: the records showed everything. It was never in my nature to go after anyone. Nursing is like that, though. Nurses will sink their teeth in you and the phrase nurses are most proud of is, "We eat our young!" I think that really speaks to the insecurities of most nurses and the overall dysfunction in the profession. Anyway, I was being pressed about Mike's work ethics or lack thereof. I recounted the incident with the suicidal patient lying for hours with nothing done. I also mentioned his lying about the cardiac monitor, the oxygen administration on the hypoxic patient, the drunk patient he let elope, etc. The list went on, and I just directed the manager to look up the charts.

As a result, Mike was called back into HR. He was placed on a probation period. Accordingly, he could not take his summer vacation. With that, Mike decided to give a two-week notice. He was now going to quit. I was sorry I was so happy to see him go.

A nurse named Patsy took his place. She said she came from a big inner-city trauma center! I thought it was going to be great. I would be working with a strong nurse again, and together I thought we could make the ER the best in the county! Man, I couldn't have been more wrong!

It was a Sunday evening and Patsy had a very ill septic patient. I was going about my business when I noticed her patient's alarms going off! The patient's blood pressure was 70! I told Patsy about it and she immediately snapped at me! She screamed, "I got it!" I've been around these nurses before. They didn't want to be told anything, and I got the message, "Back off!"

I tried to mind my own business, but after two hours of alarms I informed Patsy her patient's pressure was 40! Patsy did nothing to alert the physician! So, I went to the doctor and told him about the patient's blood pressure. I set up for a central line and helped him with the insertion. I then spiked a bag of saline, put it on a pressure bag, and began rapid infusions. I set up a CVP monitor and then mixed the Levophed, which I titrated to dial the patient's blood pressure and mean arterial pressure to normal levels. The patient was chilled, so I placed her on a Bair Hugger, which blew a blanket of warm air over her. She was so happy! As for Patsy, unknowingly, I had made an enemy for life!

Patsy brought in a patient with chest pain. Generally, with these sorts of patients we work as a team to get the patient worked up as efficiently as possible. I stepped into the room as the patient was lying on the gurney and began to place the patient on the cardiac monitor. Patsy immediately walked around to my side and pulled the EKG cables out of my hand! I was blown away. It was another clear message to back off. I left the room. You think I would've learned by now! Later, Patsy was walking a young boy into a room. He looked sick, had a fever, and reminded me of another young patient who went into V-tach and died on me years ago. I wanted to help and see the patient for myself. I walked into the room and took the patient's temperature when Patsy again came over to me and took the thermometer out of my hand! Who does that? I was now done with her!

From then on, I kept to myself as we worked our shifts. I took my patient load and read my nursing books instead of engaging with Patsy. I guess she didn't like that either. I was approached by the manager that I was giving Patsy the silent treatment! I knew things were going to get crazy, and I had to be very skilled not to get caught up in her web!

I remember one particularly crazy day. Patsy had a patient she put in a bed and walked away. His alarms were going off and I told Patsy his heart rate was 150! She began screaming, "I got it!" When I offered to help start the IV and get blood, I thought she was going to have a stroke!

A while later, the CT technician walked in and told me he had a patient in the waiting room who needed her IV taken out. I went out there, disconnected the IV, and sent the patient on her way. About an hour later, I overheard Pasty tell someone she was waiting for a CT patient to arrive. She was going to take out her IV. I then mentioned to Patsy, "Oh, they were here. I took it out."

Patsy lost it! She was screaming, "Well, thanks for telling me! I've been waiting for hours, setting hourly reminders all day!" I just looked at her as if she was crazy. It was a far cry from thanking me for taking care of it.

Wouldn't you know it, I was soon back in HR. It appeared that Patsy and I had a problem that needed to be resolved. Somehow, I was to blame. I recounted her constantly screaming at me, I identified the witnesses, I brought up the hypotensive patient. I told about her pulling the EKG leads from me, the thermometer, and the CT IV. They just looked at me. I asked them if they wanted me to mind my own business and watch her patients crash? If that's what they wanted, that's what I'd do. The manager and HR director were stupefied. I had nothing else to say. She was their problem.

A week later, Patsy had a chest pain patient who she put in a bed and left. The ER technician couldn't find her and showed me the EKG. The patient was having a huge heart attack! Patsy wasn't around, so I went in the room, started the IV, and got the doctor. While I was giving the aspirin and nitroglycerine, Patsy appeared, screaming at me that this was her patient and the doctor should speak to her if he needed anything! I just looked up at her and said, "Not now." Not 10 minutes later did this whole situation repeat itself! The patient had a racing heart beat and chest pain, and Patsy was nowhere to be found. The doctor grabbed me and I worked him up. Patsy was now psychotic, but fortunately for me her behavior was finally witnessed by the manager. He saw it all, and with that I was totally in the clear. Thank you.

Now, Patsy was still intent on frying me. I was being counseled because she felt I was looking over her shoulder and didn't trust her. I had to laugh. I unloaded. Clearly, the manager was out of his element, so I addressed everything. I told the manager I wasn't looking over her shoulder. The main station alarms were going off right in my face! I then asked, "Who leaves a patient hypotensive for two hours? Who leaves a patient with a heart rate of 150? Who walks away from active chest pain patients? Finally, who hangs a liter of normal saline on a two-year-old? You're right, I don't trust her. Do you?" He looked at me speechless. I had nothing else to say. Patsy was his problem, but I never got a response.

CHAPTER 48

REFLECTIONS THEN AND NOW

A long time ago, I was with a friend, peering out over the Pacific in search of the best surf break. I remember a brown Ford van pulling up. The driver was smoking a joint and blasting a Bob Marley tune. He was 40; he was old. At that moment, I decided I didn't want to be him. I wanted to do something with my life.

It was the aroma of garlic that got me to the door of that wonderful English woman. That's how I became a nurse. I achieved excellent grades in nursing school and, along with another student, was awarded a scholarship. Mary was a delightful young lady. We shared a lot in common: we were both a bit older than the other students, we were both married, and we both had children.

As we left our clinical one day, Mary pulled out of the hospital parking lot and was rear-ended by another automobile. Her chest then slammed against the steering wheel of her car. Mary got up out of the car and collapsed. Her aorta was torn away from her heart. She would have been a great nurse. I think of her sometimes.

Back at work, I found myself in the manager's office again. I was counseled on unresolved issues with Patsy. I wanted to laugh. I asked, "How am I to behave when she is the one constantly snapping, yelling, and screaming? What if it were me carrying on? Then what?" There was no response to that question!

I was then confronted with ignoring the ER technician who worked weekends. I took my gloves off. I began to recite how the tech slept for the first two hours of the shift and then complained about not being paid enough to work here. I recounted the time I was the only nurse in the department as two patients arrived—one for an antibiotic infusion, the other for a blood transfusion. I told the manager that I asked the technician to get the patients in a room and in a gown while I went to the lab for the blood. His response was no because he hadn't woken up yet!

I went on to talk about how I worked hard and achieved the highest grades in school. As a result, I received a number of scholarships. I asked her if they ever looked at my resume that listed the awards I had received. They weren't just scholastic but included nurse of the year awards from two hospitals and a reserve firefighter award from the city in which I once volunteered. I went on to say I take my work seriously. I asked how I am to work with a person who had an attitude like this. I told them I really couldn't, and I wouldn't. Instead, I'd pretend the tech just wasn't there. I thought the whole thing was insane. We worked in an emergency room and I was being counseled about the hurt feelings of someone who didn't even do his job? They just looked at me and said, "It's really hard to get good employees!" Yeah, but why was I in here? Why am I getting counseled? Oh, how could I forget, no one cares about nurses. After all, I've been getting punished ever since I went to school for this job!

Back in the ER, I got a young baby, 10 months old, who was in respiratory distress. He was wheezing and had intercostal retractions. His O2 saturation was also low. The baby's sister was being seen simultaneously. I triaged her, and she was fine.

I then approached the doctor and told her there were two kids in there. I pointed out that the young one was the sick one. The doctor looked at the vital signs that I took and said, "He's got a fever!"

She was talking to me like I was some ignorant loser, which is about as condescending as you could get! I just looked at her and was thinking, "Really?" I was the one who took the patient's temperature. The doctor sat on the patient for five hours. I finally went up to her with my hard hat on and said, "I know you want to send him home, but you can't. He has to be transferred and admitted." I told the doctor the last thing you want is for the patient to crash at home. The doctor was pissed. She looked up at me and said, "I don't like the way you talk to me!" The patient was transferred to the pediatric ward.

The role of a nurse is first and foremost that of a patient advocate. Still, it often comes at a cost. The cost, I recognized, was inversely proportional to the physician's competence. The better the doctor, the more grateful they would be when you alerted them to a problem. The shittier the doctor, the more hell you would have to pay. It wouldn't be so bad if the patients' lives didn't depend on it.

Now, I really believed this doctor had major issues and certainly had issues with men. She harbored a disdain for nurses, especially me. She would always be throwing her weight around and tended to act like quite the smart-ass. Still, it seemed calculated. It was just enough to jab you but leave you wondering if she was joking or if she meant it. The line was very thin. One day, for instance, I was charting. She walked by, swung her stethoscope, and struck the bony prominence of my wrist. It hurt. She said, "That's for you. You had that coming!" I still needed the job to support my family, so I continued my charting.

Not 10 minutes later, the front called for a STAT triage. I ran out and was directed to the parking lot. There, I opened the passenger door to see the driver's mother lose consciousness. She also lost her pulse. I grabbed her, put her in a wheelchair, and ran into the ER. I yelled to the clerk, "Call a code blue!" I was in the crash room and no one appeared. I struggled to get the patient on the gurney and start CPR. Still, no one was around. The technician entered and started doing CPR while I placed the defibrillator pads on the patient. I asked, "Where is everyone?" She informed me that the doctor told her not to call the code blue until she had seen the patient.

I shocked the patient as the doctor walked in while we continued CPR. I started an IV as she intubated the patient. I gave another shock and her vital signs returned. The patient was waking up and fighting the tube in her throat, so I asked for some medication to sedate her. Shortly thereafter, the patient was admitted to the ICU. Hours later she was extubated, and three days later she went home to her family. I knew a lot of doctors and a number of great ones, but sometimes I have nothing to say.

Dr. Vas pulled a shift with me the other day. I was helping him pull fluid out of a patient's chest. I got the man into position and set up the tray. Dr. Vas was about to introduce the needle and asked me if I knew why he was going over the top of the rib with his puncture. I responded, "So as not to lacerate the intercostal artery."

With that he told me, "You wasted your life. You should have been a doctor."

Dr. Vas was discharging a homeless man. The guy was a mess. But before he left, I washed the dirt off his feet, washed his face, and gave him a shave. I was also able to give him lunch and a drink. That's what I do. I'm a nurse.

CHAPTER 49

BACK AT IT

I was called in early for my shift. Turns out a nurse was assigned to work in the ICU, but there was an issue. The nursing supervisor called me explaining that the staff nurse was upset and was in tears because she had pulled the ICU shift and really expected to be working in the ER that day. Consequently, I came in early and was paid time and a half at that! I was wondering why management would cater to this behavior and not just fire the person, but it really wasn't my problem.

I walked into the unit and received report on the patient. He was an older man being treated for pneumonia and wasn't doing well. He refused intubation and was a DNR. Assisting his ventilations was the BiPAP machine. I noticed that the mask on his face was too small and fastened too tightly, so his face was becoming indented. I called the respiratory therapist and we changed the mask to one that fit. I noticed the man was dirty, so I began to clean him up. As I turned him to his side, I found he had been lying on a monitor cable that wasn't hooked up to anything and the skin on his back was broken down. I knew that though this patient was very ill, that he was going to die and his life was over, in a sense none of this really mattered. But it mattered to me. I called the nursing supervisor and told her, "Here, take a look at this!"

A while later, the man's son arrived. He stayed beside his father for most of the day. This son loved his father very much, it was palpable. Sometime near the end of the shift, the patient passed away with his loving son beside him. As I approached, the young man turned, grabbed me, and gave me a hug. As we held onto each other, he expressed his gratitude. As usual, I had to ask for certain information as to the family's wishes. I filled out the paperwork, the death papers. I walked the son out to his car. We said our goodbyes.

Walking back into the hospital, I passed the parking space where a car raced up. It was there I delivered a baby the week before. I began reflecting and thinking, nursing is the best job in the world. If you take on the responsibility of caring for people, it will carry a high demand. I was lucky to have Ms. Sue, my nursing instructor, on my shoulder all these years ensuring I do the right thing. I was even more lucky to have worked for Dr. Mack, who demanded excellence, in his flight program. Looking back to my beginning, it was Dr. Mary and Dr. Hope who really inspired me. I came to believe that nursing is a sacred profession.

Entering the hospital, I was feeling especially proud of the work I had done, proud of what I did with my time here on earth. As I was walking down the hall, I passed a patient's room. There were a few people in there. I made eye contact with a family member. Just then, I heard, "Oh, Nurse!"

ACKNOWLEDGEMENTS

To those leaders, the beacons that illuminated the way, I say thank you.

Dr. Marianne Gausche-Hill, thank you for your never-ending passion in advancing emergency care. You made me want to become a better nurse. You made me believe I could be. Dr. Hilary Bartels, it was your standards and ethics I always wanted to mirror; you were my benchmark. Dr. Jim Neiman, thank you for your brilliance and your tireless efforts in refining and improving emergency cardiac care. You were a true inspiration, you truly gave me purpose. To Dr. Jim Gude, a real professor of medicine: how I enjoyed hanging on your every word. Thank you for spreading those seeds of smiles. Dr. Gerald Lazzareschi, thank you for your kind friendship over so many years. I never tired from telling you what to do! Dr. John McDonald (RIP), thank you for your most infectious passion and for placing me on your team. You pushed me to my limits.

Where would I have been without my nurse family? Thank you from the beginning, Bill Stuehler, it really was all your fault, you ignited my fire! I'd never forget my beautiful sisters who continue to prove to me that nursing is the ultimate profession. Thank you, Deidre Allabashi, Debra Wycoff, Laurie Anderson, and Rona Hall. What a time we have had.

The list would not be complete without my show of gratitude for my days with Stacy Futer, Amy Henry, and of course you, Marcie Torres. You guys are the best of the best (NorCal)! Barry Koster, thank you for always keeping me standing. The nurses' nurse, Kathy Moix, you are truly an angel here on earth. Thank you. It was you, Silvia Mihara, you opened your door and began my journey. Thank you. I hope I made you proud.

Thank you to the crew at Paper Raven Books for guiding my hand in making this story.

To my wife, if it wasn't for you!

CPSIA information can be obtained
at www.ICGtesting.com
Printed in the USA
LVHW012350250219
608761LV00010B/220/P